HEALTH SMART CHURCH PROGRAM

Dr. Gavin's Health Guide

for African Americans

James R. Gavin III, MD, PhD
with Sherrye Landrum

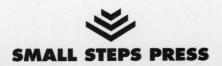

SMALL STEPS PRESS

Publisher, John Fedor; *Associate Director, Consumer Books,* Sherrye Landrum; *Editor,* Abe Ogden; *Associate Director, Book Production,* Peggy M. Rote; *Composition,* Circle Graphics; *Cover Design,* Koncept, Inc.; *Photography,* Cade Martin Photography; *Printer,* Transcontinental Printing.

Printed in Canada
1 3 5 7 9 10 8 6 4 2

Small Steps Press is an imprint of the American Diabetes Association.
Consult a health care professional before trying any of the suggestions in this publication. Small Steps Press and ADA assume no responsibility for any injury that may result from the suggestions or information in this publication.

∞ The paper in this publication meets the requirements of the ANSI Standard Z39.48-1992 (permanence of paper).

Small Steps Press titles may be purchased for business or promotional use or for special sales. To purchase this book in large quantities, or for custom editions of this book with your logo, contact Lee Romano Sequeira, Special Sales & Promotions, at the address below, or at Lees@smallstepspress.com or 703-299-2046.

Small Steps Press
1701 North Beauregard Street
Alexandria, Virginia 22311

Library of Congress Cataloging-in-Publication Data

Gavin, James R., 1945-
   Dr. Gavin's health guide for African Americans / by James R. Gavin with Sherrye Landrum.
      p. cm.
   Includes bibliographical references and index.
   ISBN 1-58040-204-6 (pbk. : alk. paper)
      1. African Americans—Health and hygiene. 2. African Americans—Diseases.
   I. Title: Health guide for African Americans. II. Landrum, Sherrye. III. Title.

RA778.4.A36G38 2004
613'.089'96073—dc22

                                                           2004041713

CONTENTS

FOREWORD

Like Dr. Martin Luther King, Jr., we in medicine and in public health also have dreams. Those dreams are to make sure that everybody in this country has access to quality health care and that disparities in health among different racial, ethnic and socioeconomic groups are eliminated. That's an extension of Dr. King's dream, but it's really critical for the future of this country.

Why? Because we are being challenged with epidemics of diseases that are life-long and responsible for lots of damage to the person who develops them. For example, obesity is an epidemic that is striking the entire population of the United States, hitting especially hard in ethnic communities and triggering serious diseases, such as diabetes, heart disease and cancer, in children and adults alike. This is the first time in the history of our country that we have seen an epidemic brought on by diet and lack of exercise. If the good life means plenty of fast food to eat and plenty of machines to do our work for us and entertain us so we don't have to get out of our chairs, well, the good life is not good for us.

Going to see the doctor is important, but it is not going to help much if you don't take charge of your own health. Humans need to eat vegetables and fruits and whole grains. Humans need to take walks after eating, and human kids need regular physical education at school and to run and play after school. If we don't do these things, our bodies and brains just don't work right—and there is nothing much your doctor or any doctor can do about it. Medical researchers are clanging the alarm bells for attention as they watch younger and younger children sliding into the cycle of obesity, diabetes, heart disease, and early death.

We can do something about this epidemic, and it doesn't take expensive drugs or surgery. We can do something about this epidemic right now, starting in our own homes with dinner tonight. It doesn't take long to prepare a healthy meal, with leftovers for lunch boxes tomorrow, but simple life choices like these will pay you back with better health in your family for generations to come.

In the case of diabetes, for example, we know that by changing lifestyles we can prevent the onset of 50 to 60% of type 2 diabetes, which is 90% of the diabetes we see in this country. This is good news for millions of people, more and more of them younger than 20 years old. We also know we could prevent complications like kidney disease and blindness and the need for lower limb amputation if we find them early and treat them. You must take responsibility for your own health and work closely with health care professionals to get the care you need. And you must take better care of yourself.

This book can show you several ways to make vast and sweeping changes in your lives, if you are willing to try. Hopefully, it will encourage you to search for new ways that you and your family can live well and be well at the same time.

David Satcher, M.D., Ph.D.
Former Surgeon General of the United States
Director, Center for Primary Care
Morehouse School of Medicine

INTRODUCTION

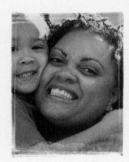

It has always been the hope of adults that it will be the children that save us. However, in the 21st century, African American and Latino children are falling ill with diseases that 15 years ago only middle-aged or elder adults developed. Children with the chronic, crippling, and debilitating diseases of adulthood, such as high blood pressure, obesity, heart disease, and diabetes are our worst nightmare. And that nightmare is coming true. One in every four children is obese, which causes a long list of serious health problems. One in every three children will develop diabetes and some form of heart disease. We must do something about this now. Fortunately, we can do something about this.

Even though we grown-ups know that we need to eat better and exercise more, which is the simple cure for most illnesses, we don't do it for ourselves. Sadly, our children are following too closely in our footsteps. Look around you. They eat the fried foods and the fast foods and drink sugary sodas in grown-up sized servings that are too big even for grown-ups. Like us, they ride and sit instead of walking or running. They do not engage in vigorous physical activity, the kind that tones and strengthens their bodies and develops their coordination. They don't play outside anymore, not even at school.

The plain truth is that we have an awful lot of people, young and old, "digging their graves with their teeth," as my grandmama used to say.

With all of this grim information, it's easy to get discouraged. If your grandmother is in a wheelchair from an amputation caused by diabetes and she's on dialysis, you and your children may feel that you are doomed to get diabetes and the same problems she has. If your whole family is overweight, you may feel that you cannot change that. But you can. Your grandparents didn't have the tools and the information for prevention and treatment that are available to you now. When your grandparents were first suffering, we in the medical community didn't have the knowledge and awareness about many of these diseases. You, on the other hand, have decades of research and advancements at your disposal. You have the power to lose weight and to help your children lose weight. You have the power to do what you need to do.

The fact is that no one is doomed here. You and your children do not have to go down the same path as the generation before and end up on dialysis or have a heart attack. You don't have to die young. You and I can do something about this epidemic in America. We can help those who are already ill, and we can prevent any more from falling ill. And along the way, we will become healthier, too.

But this isn't just going to happen on its own. You and I are the only ones who can do the things that will save the children—and ourselves. Doctors can't fix this for us. No pill can conquer this challenge. Only we can save ourselves.

Do I have your attention?

I want you to help create a new world, starting with yourself. This book can show you how to get things going. Let's put the spotlight where it belongs—on being well. I want you and your children to live long and healthy lives. I want you to have a rich quality of life, even with opportunities for love and joy. This is my goal as your family doctor, my offer of support as your personal consultant on your family's health.

We Are Living Ourselves to Death

The health challenge that faces every American, regardless of ethnic background, is deadly serious, and it comes from having too much to eat and too little exercise. Because you are also African American or Latino, your risk of developing serious diseases is two to three times higher. You cannot afford to ignore what is happening, and you can't let fear stop you in your tracks. You need to recognize your risk and then take the steps to reduce your chances of catastrophic health problems, such as kidney disease, heart disease, hypertension, diabetes, stroke, and more.

What Is Your Risk for Serious Health Problems?

- If you are more than 30 pounds overweight or your child is in the 80% of weight for his age, you're both at risk.
- If you have high blood pressure, you're at risk.
- If you have high cholesterol, you're at risk.
- If you have diabetes, you're at risk.
- If you or your child smoke cigarettes, you're at risk.
- If you have all of these conditions—and too many people do—then you are a walking heart attack waiting to explode. Even if you're only 12 years old.

The Beautiful People

People buy lots of magazines and books, the covers plastered with impossibly beautiful people, in the hopes that the secret answer to their problem will be hidden inside. The secret to weight loss; the secret to lowering blood pressure; the secret to lowering cholesterol; the secret to staying sexy forever; the secret to building muscles; the secret to burning all the fat you don't want on your body; the secret to long life and happiness. Well, let me share a simple truth with you—the answers you're looking for aren't secrets. You get healthy by using common sense and going back to doing what comes naturally. This common sense method does not sell magazines and videos, so you don't hear a lot about it. But take my word for it, common sense is the surest way to help you change your life and save your children's lives, too.

What we have in America today is an energy crisis. We have too much energy going into our bodies and not enough activity to use up the energy that we eat. Look around. Is your child sitting next to you on the couch? Lying on the floor? Parked in front of a video game? Don't yell at him to go outside and play. Take him by the hand and both of you go outside and be active together. Throw a Frisbee or a baseball. Jump rope. Go down to the school and walk around the track. Then shoot some baskets and swing on the monkey bars. Put some life back into your life.

Remember that children know very well when you tell them to do one thing and then you do another. Earn their respect. *You* do as you say.

The Mystery and the Miracle of Energy

Of course, all of this talk of being active is easy to say and not as easy to do. You may feel that you don't have the energy to get up and do anything. If you are overweight or your blood sugar is high, you feel wiped out. You have plenty of fuel but no energy. That's the mystery of energy. The miracle of energy is that once you get up and start moving, you get more energy. You jumpstart your motor by moving, and if you keep moving every day, you can surprise yourself with how much energy you have and how good you feel. In fact, I have often said to patients that once you start a regular program of physical activity your body seems to do a flip-flop. Instead of feeling bad when you exercise, you get to a point where the only time you feel good is when you exercise. It is a good and rewarding habit to develop. Try it.

Why do you feel so good? Physical activity lowers your blood pressure, lowers your blood sugar, and burns food so it is not stored as fat. Exercise releases powerful natural chemicals (endorphins) in your body that relieve pain and make you feel good. Your body feels better because it's working the way God made it to work. Common sense, see?

You eat food so your body can burn it for fuel to get energy to think, to move, to grow, and to heal. We measure that potential energy in food as calories. Driving and watching a TV or a computer are activities that don't burn many calories. In fact, they take the active right out of the word "activities." You're not burning a lot of fuel just sitting there. Unfortunately, instead of eating just a little to match our actual fuel usage, we usually eat enough food to run a marathon or climb mountains. Is the truth that you don't even climb the stairs at work? Most people drive around extra minutes in the parking lot just trying to find a space 10 yards closer to the entrance. We have to stop this! Park in the back of the lot, walk the extra distance, and burn off some of that extra fuel. Your body needs it.

What Is Happening to Our Children?

In the past 20 years, the entire food balance has shifted in the United States. We have easy access to too much food, especially fast food. Burgers, fries, sodas, crispy chickens, and extra large burritos are everywhere, so we eat them in excess quantities. This too-much-of-a-bad-thing way of eating is particularly bad in our children. Why? Our children watch, read, and hear those 25 billion dollars worth of food advertisements aimed directly at them. Have you noticed these advertisements are not for low-calorie vegetables and fruit? This is one of the reasons why our kids drink too many sweetened beverages and eat too much processed food. But the more important reason is that these are the foods we choose to let our children eat.

Even babies eat too much. It's okay to carry a bottle with you, but if you let her carry it, she's going to drink it. Babies don't need to be eating all the time—not any more than you do. Even juice and milk can start the babies on the road to obesity early. If your baby wants a bottle for comfort between meals, put water in it. It's good to develop a taste for water early in life.

On top of poor food choices and an enormous calorie intake, children are much less active today than they were in the past. Too much time is spent (about 3 to 4 hours on average) planted in front of a screen of some kind. Their levels of physical activity are way out of step with the amount of food they're cramming into their bodies. The result is a lot of extra calories being stored as fat.

Fuel Economy: We Get Great Gas Mileage

It turns out, there's a reason so much of the extra food we and our kids are eating is stored as fat. Many of us have what is called a "thrifty gene" (it's really a cluster of genes) that protected our ancestors in time of famine or too little food. We get a lot of miles out of the food we eat. When people with the thrifty gene eat too much food every day for years, we become obese. Then we get all the diseases that go along with being obese.

To keep this from happening, you want to put only premium fuel in your body, just as you do in your car. What's premium fuel? Fruits and vegetables, whole grains, skim milk products, nuts and beans, and lean meat. You probably already knew that. You probably have also ignored it. Even though our markets are full of fruits and vegetables here in the United States, only one person in five, young or old, eats their suggested five to nine vegetables and fruits every day. Wouldn't you like to be that one wise person?

Do you put fruits and vegetables in the lunches you and your spouse take to work? How about the lunches your kids take to school? Probably not, and more than likely, your kids are looking to other easily accessible sources of food. Nowadays, schools have vending machines for hungry kids to visit. Across the country, 78% of high schools have vending machines, as do 14% of elementary schools. In fact, vending machines have become a way for schools to raise money through an agreement with the vending machine companies.

Are vending machines a good place for your kids to shop for their meals? What are the choices made available to our kids? Fresh fruit, fruit juice, carrot sticks, and whole grain muffins? Not really. The usual choices are items like regular sodas, chips, cookies, and candy. As a result, many kids in school are sometimes drinking 2 to 3 sodas a day and skipping the cafeteria lunch unless it comes from a fast food restaurant. Is that a good lunch? In a year, these 2 to 3 sodas for lunch add up to as many as 500–700 cans of soda. That's a lot of sugar and a lot of empty calories (see the box "Liquid Calories"). Add the sugar in the cookies and candy and you can see why our kids are overweight. It's better to chew calories than to drink them. We weren't designed to live on chips, cookies, and sodas, but that is what our children are doing. It's not just the kids. Every year, we grownups are eating 150 pounds of sweeteners, 54 gallons of soda, and 200 pounds of refined grains (white pasta and rice). We can make better food choices.

Liquid Calories

There doesn't seem to be a single place in this country where you can't buy soda. Work, school, restaurants, convenience stores, grocery stores, even electronics stores; it's everywhere. So what's the impact of this? Let's say you drink three cans of soda a day. At 150 calories a can (at least) that's 450 calories—more than a McDonald's quarter-pound hamburger, and about 1/4 of the total calories a person should eat in an entire day! And those are empty calories with almost no nutritional value. Over a year, those three regular sodas a day add up to 1,095 cans, or 164,250 calories. That's like eating 1,175 drumsticks of fried chicken on top of what you're already eating! Keep in mind that these are 12-ounce cans of soda, just about the smallest portion you can buy. If you get a soda at a convenience store or fast food restaurant, it's more than likely going to be around 32 ounces. Drinking three of these is like eating an entire half of a pepperoni pizza! Which would you rather have? My advice—cut out the soda and drink water or tea. If you are going to drink soda, just drink less. Instead of the super-size monster, get the small portion and actually enjoy what you're drinking instead of gulping it down. All of those calories are adding up, why not enjoy them?

Use It or Store It as Fat?

Now let's look at your child's opportunities to burn calories
in school. Thinking uses some calories, but not nearly as
many calories as kids are taking in. Physical Education (PE),
or gym class, was required every day for all students in the
1970s. Now only one in four kids have gym class, and that's
just two days a week. To round out this sad picture, research
shows that in a 45-minute PE class, kids only actually move a
total of about six minutes.

Is this helping our children? Instead of a 45-minute class
that's 39 minutes of milling around, students should start
every day by walking around the track or circling the playground eight times. This would be better for our kids and
good for the teachers, too. Teachers could divide classes or
homerooms into two teams (for example a red and a blue
team) so everybody in the school is on one team or the other,
say the Reds and Blues. Keep track of how far each team
walks on a big board in the hall, so the Reds can see how
they're doing against the Blues. It's fun and can motivate
your child to walk. You would do everyone a lot of good if
you suggest it at the next PTO meeting. Let's put activity
back into the school day for the good of us all.

If you talk with the principal about this, you may be told
that PE has been cut to give kids more time to study. Here's
your answer: Research proves that kids who are active and
physically fit think better and do better on tests. Fitness
equals better testing scores and better testing scores equal
better opportunities for the school. This is another reason
why physical activity is so important to our children. It's
good for their minds as well as their bodies.

Remember what I said earlier about this problem not fix-
ing itself? This is part of what I meant. To stem the tide of
this epidemic you are going to have to speak up—at home, at
school, at work. You need to be involved in your children's

lives and to find out what they are doing—and not doing—that is having an enormous effect on how they feel now and how long and how well they will live. The whole family must get involved if we are to save the children.

The Short Course

To get yourself in good shape, you need to take four steps. Follow these steps, and you're well on your way to a longer, happier, and healthier life.

Step 1

Step 1 is to know your risk for getting ill. Medical science has the answer—your risk level is high. That's the bad news. The good news is that you can do things every day to make your risk low.

Step 2

Step 2 is to learn what affects your health. We know the answer to this one, too.

What changes your weight?

Food, physical activity, stress, and medication.

What changes diabetes?

Food, physical activity, stress, and medication.

What changes your blood pressure?

Food, physical activity, stress, and medication.

What changes your cholesterol?

Food, physical activity, stress, and medication.

What changes your heart health?

Food, physical activity, stress, and medication.

Got the picture? Your doctor can prescribe a useful medication if you need one, but medication comes last—after you have done all you can for your body. What you eat, what activities you do, and how you deal with stress all have a huge impact on your health. These are the three keys to better health that you can use right now, with no equipment, at no extra cost.

Step 3

Step 3 is to follow my simple prescription for how to change your health:

Give yourself TLC (therapeutic lifestyle changes).

Start low, go slow. How can you change your approach to food? Eat less than now. Start at your next meal. Learn which foods give you the nutrition you need and which foods don't. Add a healthier food, such as a fruit or vegetable to each of your meals. Drink five glasses of water a day.

How can you add physical activity to your life? Do more than you're doing now. Start the next time you park your car. You don't need to join a gym. Park at the far end of the parking lot on purpose. Don't ride around looking for a spot that's a few feet closer to the entrance. The spot you want is in the very back. If you're in a multistory building, and you have to change floors, take the stairs. If you travel through airports a lot, walk up the escalators. People stand there like it's a carnival ride. They're still stairs folks and they invite you to make use of them. Come on, get moving!

Step 4

Step 4 is to recognize the power of what you do. Exercise is good stuff. It does wonderful things. Eating good is just as great. Fruits, vegetables, whole grains, nuts, and olive oil provide your body with the right fuel to do all it has to do. These foods were put here on earth not just for us to taste and to enjoy, but to keep us healthy in body and mind. This isn't religion; this is common sense.

My Common Sense "Secrets" to Being Well

- Take a 30-minute walk every day.
- Eat at least 3 vegetables and 2 fruits every day.
- Drink 6 to 8 glasses of water every day. More if you're playing hard and sweating a lot.
- Smile, and smile often.
- Stop smoking.
- Ask your doctor if you should take a baby aspirin every day.
- (Remember that if you do these first 6 things every day, you're golden.)
- When you're learning something new, take baby steps and laugh when you fall down.
- Eat good food. You deserve the delicious taste of real food.
- Get enough sleep—you may need 8 to 9 hours to feel rested and well.
- Figure out how to lighten your heart, and laugh more often.
- Hug someone (it's better if you actually know them).
- One glass of wine or beer with dinner is good for adult health. If you can't stop at one, make a toast with a

glass of tea instead and take a walk after dinner to count your blessings.

- Read books, magazines, newspapers, internet articles, food labels, and anything else that can help you choose well and live a richer, fuller life.

- Try to meet people of all ages, and be curious, so you will have some good stories to tell.

- Have and enjoy good conversations.

- Know good people. If your family is made up of cranky folks, find some cheerful friends, and bring laughter home with you.

- Give your children helpful jobs to do, so their lives also have meaning. Let them help shop for food and prepare it. Let them help clean up afterward, too.

- If something isn't working for you, change it. You have that power.

- Find the right place and the right fit for God and worship in your life. People who go to church actually live longer, on average, than those who don't.

- Focus on wellness, not illness. Small acts translate to hope and tremendous outcomes.

Enjoy Life

This is my most important "secret" of all. We share a multicultural background that we blend into something unique in each of our families. We embrace our love of family, church, food, and music. We must also embrace, and enjoy, these challenges to our health that we share as a result of our genes and our lifestyle choices.

The keys to enjoying life are good food, good conversation, good people, and good music. The first three seem obvious, but the last one seems to often get neglected. If you listen to good music (and what's good is your call) every day, and you dance around the kitchen or the living room to three or four songs, then you have been active for 10 minutes. Your heart rate is up, your face is flushed and glowing, and your mood is improved, too. Dancing is not just for young folks or weddings. Dancing and singing are healthy activities you need to do every day.

Music can change your mental outlook and your emotions, too. You know which songs make you feel like smiling and tapping your feet, and which songs make you sad. You know how emotion can tie up your energy so you don't feel like doing anything. Play the music that makes you move. Use your common sense.

I love to sing and, fortunately, God gave me a voice that people enjoy listening to. But it doesn't matter if you can sing well, just do it. Singing counts as physical activity, especially when you put your whole self into the song. Just recently I attended a Patti LaBelle concert and witnessed up close the amount of energy expended by this remarkably talented woman, a woman who has taken charge of her diabetes. If you need help to get moving—whether you're walking or sweeping the floor—put on music or sing a song that fires you up. Encourage yourself and have fun, too. Use the power you already have.

Resources

General

First and foremost we must learn to read. If you're reading this paragraph, literacy is obviously not a problem for you. But what about a loved one? Whether it's for a child or an adult, reading is a great gift to give. A person needs to be able to read prescription labels and the care plan that a doctor works out. Your parents or grandparents or children need to be able to read about health research and what it means for them.

A great way to learn is by watching a video. Take a look at *Phonics and Fables* and *Ready for Adult Phonics* at: *www.shopPBS.com*
Or call 1-800-645-4727 to learn more.

You might see if your local library or adult learning center (often in the local high schools) has these videos for you to check out for free.

We also need to be involved with the legislation and government activities that affect our health. Contact your local representatives to Congress at: *www.congress.org*

Online

We need to start using the resources available to us. One of the biggest resources available to us is the Internet. Search engines are websites that help you find information on any topic. Some of the best known ones are: *www.google.com* and *www.askjeeves.com*

I'm sure you'll find others. Check with the librarian at your local library. Most public libraries have computers available for you to use, and many offer classes in how to use the Internet.

A good general information website for community improvement can be found at:
www.helpyourcommunity.org

A good online destination that includes a resource library, a kitchen and nutrition center, a mind-body room, a weekly support group chat and a monthly drop-in group can be found at:
www.wellness-community.org

A website designed to help strengthen marriages and friendships, raise loving and resilient children, deepen faith, expand creativity, develop a healthier body image, and discover greater purpose and meaning in life is at:
www.thelearningplaceonline.com

Associations

National Library of Medicine
8600 Rockville Pike
Bethesda, MD 20894
888-346-3656
www.nlm.nih.gov

The Office of Minority Health Resource Center (OMHRC)
This center distributes information on cancer, heart disease and stroke, diabetes, homicide, suicide, unintentional injuries, HIV/AIDS, infant mortality, substance abuse, and a host of other subjects. All services are free, phone lines are open from 9 A.M. to 5 P.M. Eastern Time, Monday through Friday, to help callers in English or Spanish.

P.O. Box 37337
Washington, D.C. 20013-7337
www.omhrc.gov

National Urban League
120 Wall Street
New York, NY 10005
212-558-5300
www.nul.org

The Children's Defense Fund
25 E Street, NW
Washington, D.C. 20001
202-628-8787
www.childrensdefense.org

National Medical Association
1012 Tenth Street, NW
Washington, D.C. 20001
202-347-1895
www.nmanet.org

Public Health Foundation
1220 L Street, NW, Suite 350
Washington, D.C. 20005
202-898-5600
www.phf.org

Office on Smoking and Health
Centers for Disease Control and Prevention
Publications Catalog, Mail Stop K-50
4770 Buford Highway, NE
Atlanta, GA 3034103724
800-CDC-1311 (800-232-1311)
www.cdc.gov/tobacco

American Sickle Cell Anemia Association
10300 Carnegie Avenue
Cleveland, OH 44106
216-229-8600
www.ascaa.org

Sickle Cell Disease Association of America
200 Corporate Pointe
Suite 495
Culver City, CA 90230-8727
800-421-8453
www.sicklecelldisease.org

Center for Medicare and Medicaid Services
Center for Medicare Management
7500 Security Boulevard
Baltimore, MD 21244
800-MEDICARE (800-633-4227)
www.medicare.gov

National Caucus and Center on Black Aged, Inc.
1220 L Street, NW
Suite 800
Washington, D.C. 20005
202-637-8400
www.ncba-aged.org

African American Family Services Resource Center
2616 Nicollet Avenue, South
Minneapolis, MN 55408
612-871-7878
www.aafs.net

100 Black Men of America, Inc.
An organization committed to the empowerment of the
African American community based on: respect for family,
spirituality, justice, and integrity. The focus for the future is

on mentoring and education, challenges to youth, health and
wellness, anti-violence, and economic development.
141 Auburn Avenue
Atlanta, GA 30303
1-800-598-3411
www.100blackmen.org

National Coalition of 100 Black Women
38 West 32nd Street
Suite 1610
New York, NY 10001
212-947-2196
www.ncbw.org/about/home.html

1

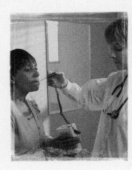

DOCTORS, RESEARCH, AND YOU

Most folks don't mind going to the doctor if they expect the news to be good. The maternity ward is a pretty happy place, by and large. But lots of people don't go to the doctor because they're afraid they're going to hear bad news. If you're one of these people, let me ask you to consider this "bad news" in another light. A serious illness discovered during a routine physical for school or work is not bad news. This is "thank goodness you found it early" news. You want to know if something is threatening your health and you want to know as early as possible so you have time to do all you can to stop it. Most of the diseases that affect us can be effectively treated, even cured, if we start early enough.

Another reason people don't go to the doctor is because they haven't done what the doctor asked them to do. Guess what? Your body isn't fooled. Are you trying to fool yourself? Why are you trying to fool yourself? What do you have to gain from that? Find out what is more important to you than your health, because you really need the answer to that question. It's the only way you can move on to making better choices for yourself.

Doctors: Your Technical Consultant

For hundreds of years, doctors have been attacking every disease we could find. We have succeeded in treating or preventing most of the acute diseases, such as appendicitis, polio, and mumps. We've reached a higher level of health than ever before. So we are all living longer lives. But now, we are living long enough to develop the diseases that doctors cannot cure, chronic diseases like diabetes and arthritis that a patient takes home and lives with for the rest of her life. This means that the responsibility has moved from us, the doctors, to you, the patient. We can't simply give you a vaccine. We can't simply write you a prescription. These are diseases and conditions that are a part of your daily life. You own these diseases now.

We health care professionals have become something new. We have become the technical advisors for you, the person who actually has the problem. I can tell you what I have learned from research and from my training and experience, information that can help you live better with diabetes or heart disease or other chronic conditions. But my power ends there. I have information for you. I can support you. I can tell you what your risks for illness are. I can do the tests and tell you what they show about your health now. I can help you make informed choices about what to do next. I can tell you where to find extra help. But I cannot make the choices for you. Only you can take care of you. And if you don't do it, who can?

What Do You Need from Your Doctor?

You need health care for your illnesses. However, different illnesses require different levels and types of health care. If you have a sore throat, that's an easy visit. We look in your throat, culture it for strep, and write you a prescription for an antibiotic if you need it. This is medicine that everybody likes. It's clean, quick, and everybody goes home happy. If you have a chronic disease, however, one that does not have a simple cure, then the office visit is not so quick and easy. You may have several lab tests, blood and urine, to check on how your body is doing. You may talk over new or long-lasting symptoms. You need good advice to help you make daily health choices. But the fact is that most doctors have about five to ten minutes to spend with you—no matter how good or bad your insurance is.

Your doctor is busy and has to see and treat many different diseases. This means you need to take some extra steps to educate yourself about your own. If you know what is important about your condition, you'll ask the right questions. You'll know what the test results mean for you.

Know what you want from the doctor or nurse before you go in—prepare for the meeting. If you go without writing down your questions, you are not going to get answers. Study yourself. What foods do you like? Do you ever take a walk? Are you sleeping well? Do you have good friends that you see often? Have you recently been exposed to any illnesses? What health problem is worrying you? What do you want to know? Where do you think you can start to make a healthy change in your lifestyle?

Knowledge Is Key

The world is full of experts. You can find them in newspapers, magazines, on TV shows, in books like this. Some of these "experts" are in your family or in the neighborhood. Some of them may say things that make sense to you. Some of them may spout utter nonsense, but until you learn more about how your body works and what it means to be healthy, you won't know that. You have a body; it is wise to learn more about it. You have to read the instruction manual for a car or a computer to use it—why not for your body, too?

The human body is an absolute miracle. Its needs are simple, despite what advertisements say. Talk with your doctor, nurse educator, and dietitian. Read books. Look into some dependable health and wellness websites, such as the government National Institutes of Health websites (*www.nih.gov*). After awhile, you'll be able to distinguish between what is dangerous or silly and what might work for you.

A Word about Research

You can read about the latest research in every newspaper and magazine in America almost every day. This news sells papers. Some of the reports can be helpful, and some just get you excited for no reason. A research study should be carefully designed and include a large group of people. If the research in the news article was a two-month study of 19 people, there's not yet enough information to apply it to everyone else in the world. If you hear about research from the Nurses Health Study or the Diabetes Control and Complications Trial (DCCT)—both of which studied thousands of people over 10 years or more—then you can be more confident that the results will hold true for most people and probably for you.

Be especially skeptical with books that announce great, brand new scientific discoveries in the book itself. This is not the usual way for credible scientific findings to be published. Books are reviewed and often edited by smart people, but not subjected to scientific peer review. Anyone who can find a willing publisher can get his views published. That does not make it good science or sound medicine.

Magazines, like *Health*, *Self*, *Time*, and *Newsweek*, collect the latest research and pepper you with it. Sometimes they talk about research that sounds a little far-fetched; usually something that talks about quick results without any work on your part. Most of the time, though, they reiterate sensible health information that's been proven in study after study, such as the benefits of daily walks and eating more fruits and vegetables. And actually, your common sense would agree that these are healthy actions for you to take. Deep down, you know what is healthy and you know what is a bunch of nonsense. But you don't walk every day, and you don't like any vegetables but fried potatoes. When are you going to start taking advantage of the information you already know?

How to Talk to Your Doctor

- Know what your questions are beforehand. Write them down in between office visits. Call about the scary ones, save the others for face-to-face time. Don't be embarrassed. This is your time with your private consultant, use your time together well. Since serious health issues can trigger some powerful emotions, try not to miss what is actually being said. If you get upset, that's okay, but be sure to get clear answers to your questions. If you need to, bring a tape recorder and turn it on so you can listen to the answers again at home. Bring a friend or a loved one as an extra set of ears. If you don't get helpful answers or advice that you can use, you may need to change doctors. Try to find one that will work with you.

How to Talk to Your Doctor (*continued*)

- Be honest. This is extremely important. Be honest with yourself and then with your doctor. Use plain language and get to the point. If you don't tell your doctor the truth about what you eat or how much you exercise or whether you smoke or drink, your health isn't that important to you anyway, so what are you doing at the doctor's office?
- Remember that what your doctor says is not the almighty truth. Would you rather get advice from family or friends than a doctor? Do you surf the Internet to get medical information? That's okay. It is a good idea to get a second—or a third—opinion. In fact, it is your responsibility to find out all you can about your health, so you can make decisions that work for you. You'll be able to give other people better advice if they develop an illness, too. You need to know your risks, your choices, the consequences of the choices, and the toolkits you can use to be well.
- Don't panic. Talk with your doctor about how to get started on your new healthy lifestyle and try not to be overwhelmed. Becoming healthy is just a new way of walking over familiar ground. Start low. Go slow. At your next meal, eat less. When you park your car, park at the back of the parking lot. Take the stairs today. Do it again tomorrow. Be proud of what you do.

Changes: The Only Constant Is Change

On the road to wellness, you're going to need to make a lot of changes along the way to reach the new life you want to lead. But making changes are hard. You've lived your entire life one way; you don't know anything else. Changes need to be examined and discussed, and they need to be gradual, or they're not going to happen at all.

When your doctor tells you that you need a new drug or to change drugs, talk over a plan so you can see how that change is going to work in your life. If it isn't going to work, tell your doctor why. If you can't afford the drug, or you won't take it, then say so.

If you don't think you can walk for 45 minutes a day, say so. Then you can discuss some things you can do to build up to 45 minutes. Or you can discuss other activities that will be easier on your joints. Know what your goal is before you leave the office. Do you know how to get there? Is the goal reasonable? Can you break it down into four steps? Can you succeed at the first step in the next month?

Why is it necessary to ask questions and discuss your behavior and personal wishes and daily schedule and demands on your time and money? Because you have to take the information doctors give you about taking care of the human body and adjust it to fit what you are willing to do. Changing daily habits is not easy to do, especially if you are not ready to do it, or can't see why you should do it.

Hopefully in this book you can find lots of reasons to think about changing to healthier behaviors. Some of the positive results of making these changes can be measured in laboratory tests and on the scale. The positive results that will change your daily life, such as having the energy and the focus to create and play and enjoy new things, only you can measure. The key to whether or not you will make changes is how much pleasure you get from taking better care of yourself. You may have to overturn years of negative thinking of yourself as powerless, so you can see what you can really do. You are worth the effort.

As David M. Spero, BSN, RN, has pointed out, "you want to make your life better, not harder. For most people, life is hard enough already." Here are some questions he suggests that you ask yourself:

1. What do you need most now? What do you want right now?
2. What about this is giving you the most trouble?

3. Is there something you'd like that your condition prevents you from doing?
4. What would make your life better or easier, or better for others?
5. In what ways would you like to feel better?
6. What would make you excited about getting out of bed in the morning?
7. What makes you feel happy or energized, and how can you get more of it?
8. What makes your life miserable, and how could that be changed?
9. What gives your life meaning? What gives you a sense of purpose?
10. What are the most important things in your life now?
11. What makes you feel useful or connected? If none, how would you like to be useful or connected?

These questions can help you develop positive health, fitness, and life goals that will motivate you to keep on making changes to take better care of yourself.

Once you have some good reasons to make a change, it helps to have an action plan. Choose a goal that is within your reach. Be specific. Instead of saying, "I'm going to lose weight," break your goal down into simple steps, such as "I'm going to eat fast food at lunch only once this week. I will pack a lunch the other four days. I'm going to treat myself to some tasty new lunches, with vegetables and fruits and lean meats." That's enough details to give you a clear picture of what you need to do. If you are pretty confident you can follow through with your plan, then go for it.

You also need to give some thought to what hurdles might get in your way. Once you've identified everything that might get you off track with this goal, what can you do to slip around these barriers to your success?

Don't try to make too many changes at once. Make one at a time. Start low, go slow. Make a list of your strengths and use them. Where have you succeeded in the past? Can you build on that success? Believe in yourself. And enjoy the folks that believe in you, too. See Chapter 4. The Power of Emotion for more on making changes.

Prescription Drugs

A lot of people are prescribed medicine without knowing why they need to take it. Prescription drugs are expensive, you should always know what you're taking and why. For chronic diseases, you're probably taking medicine because your levels—blood sugar, cholesterol, blood pressure—are high. If so, then it is wise to take the medicine you've been prescribed to get the levels back to normal and lower the risks to your health.

But medicine doesn't have to do everything by itself. While the pills are working for you, you can also start eating more nutritious foods and walking. In three months these changes in your lifestyle may be enough to get your levels to normal, and maybe you can stop taking the pills—or at least cut back on the dose.

What to Ask about Drugs

Whenever you go to the doctor, take all your medications with you in a bag, so he or she can see them. Include any vitamin supplements or herbs as well, because they are as powerful as drugs and can interact with your other medications. Once a year, review these medications with the doctor. Ask:

1. Do I still need this?
2. Do I still need to take this same dosage or to take it so often?

When your doctor prescribes a new drug for you, ask:

1. Why do I need this drug?
2. When do I take it and how often? For example, you may not be able to take a drug three times a day, and if you say so, your doctor may know of another drug you take once a day that will work as well. You won't know unless you ask.
3. How long before the drug takes effect?
4. When can I stop taking it?
5. How does it interact with my other drugs? Tell your doctor if you are taking vitamin supplements, herbs, or an over-the-counter medication—especially if you are going to have surgery.
6. What side effects might I have with this new drug?
7. Do you have any free samples or can you give me a smaller prescription to try it out? When your prescription goes out of date, throw it in the trash. Don't give it to someone else who may have a bad reaction to the drug.

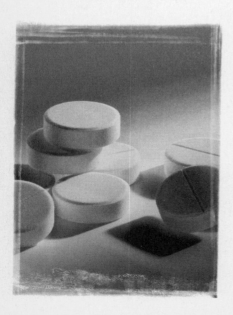

Cheap Drugs

You may have heard that prescription drugs can be bought on the Internet, and they're cheaper. Buyer beware. Go to the site *www.Pharmacy Checker.com* and check out the ratings of any pharmacy website before you buy. (Like I mentioned in the Resources section at the back of the Introduction, you can go to the library and use their computer if you do not have one of your own.) Any online pharmacy that lets you order medicine without a prescription or through a phone or e-mail consultation should be avoided. Most of the sites in Canada are closely regulated and won't let you self-prescribe. Only use a company that asks you to fax or mail your prescription. The site should be licensed by a pharmacy board. They must promise to protect your medical and credit card information, too. The site should give a street address and phone number that you can call with problems.

A safer and equally cheap alternative to online prescriptions is mail order. See if this is an option with your current health insurance. You can generally save the most money by ordering a several-month supply.

One thing to consider when drug shopping on the Internet or through the mail is the personal service you'll be sacrificing. If your local pharmacist usually tracks all your prescriptions and talks with you about interactions and side effects, you lose this gatekeeper with an online order. This could be a problem. Is it worth the extra money to get this professional advice?

Benefits Check Up Online

If you have a problem affording the drugs prescribed for you, there is help on the Internet. One of the best sites on the web, *www.BenefitsCheckUpRx.com*, tracks the 240 programs that offer assistance with drug costs, including 30 state-funded pharmacy programs and drug company assistance programs (there are about 120 right now), which generally have no age or income requirements. Also on the site are drug-discount cards that are free to consumers and must provide at least a 20% discount.

You will need to supply information about your prescription drugs. There is a pull-down menu of drug names, but many are similar, so be sure you have the correct names. You will also need to supply information about your yearly income. Most people qualify for at least one of the programs, so check it out.

If you don't have a computer, you can call toll free 1-800-677-1116. This is an eldercare locator, but they should have computer access and be able to help you.

So What's the Point of All This?

If anything, I hope this chapter showed that the responsibility of your personal well-being lies with one person—you. It's your responsibility to use the health care system for you. You are the one who should lead the conversation with your doctor to get the information that you need. If you don't understand, ask for more details. To make it easier, ask yourself these questions.

1. What do you need from your doctor?
2. What do you expect from your doctor?
3. Are the two answers the same or are they different? Are your expectations unrealistic? What should you get from your doctor?

I wish that all of us could have a health care provider who is wise, honest, and funny. That's a goal to work toward, but at the very least, you need a doctor who is community oriented, trustworthy, and easy to talk to. Your doctor should treat your whole being, not just your body.

Now having said all this, I must also say that we health care professionals don't have all the answers. We cannot solve your problems for you. The coach never carries the ball. You're playing the game, and you are here to learn a great deal about yourself. It might help to remember that there are no failures, only learning experiences. Get some.

How to Be the Best Patient

- Understand your health risks.
- Talk to your doctor about what to do about your risks.
- Get a physical exam and lab tests at least once a year.
- If you have an illness, find out what to do to manage it.
- Eat well, sleep well, walk more, laugh more.
- Take good care of your self.

Resources

Online

The Future of Family Medicine Project
www.futurefamilymed.org

The American Academy of Family Physicians
www.AAFP.org

The Robert Graham Center is an organization devoted to bringing a family practice and primary care perspective to health legislation in all levels of government.
www.graham-center.org

Associations

**National Center for Complementary
and Alternative Medicine Clearinghouse**
P.O. Box 7923
Gaithersburg, MD 20898
888-644-6226
http://nccam.nih.gov

Books

Diabetes Burnout, by William Polonsky, PhD. American Diabetes Association, 1999.

The Art of Getting Well: A Five-Step Plan for Maximizing Health When You Have a Chronic Illness, by David Spero, BSN, RN. Hunter House, 2002. You can also visit *www.art-of-getting-well.com*.

Cancer as a Turning Point, by Lawrence LeShan. Dutton, 1989.

Six Pillars of Self-Esteem, by Nathaniel Branden. Bantam, 1994.

The Physician Within, by Cathy Feste. Henry Holt and Company, 1993.

2

REAL FOOD

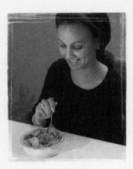

Get over all the rules. Just eat better.

—Tim Patton, MA, MPH, RD

Somehow, it seems like eating healthy has become really complicated. Between the thousands of magazine articles, weight-loss products, and fad diets, it can feel like the process of eating right is only slightly less intricate than an advanced chemistry class. Well, I'm here to tell you that it's not that complex. There is only one healthy way to eat, and the foods that are good for you are good for most everyone.

What Is Good Eating?

In general, good eating is eating good foods sensibly. Sounds easy, doesn't it? We all know it isn't that easy, but I can tell you it's not nearly as hard as we make it. Start with the first part.

Good Food

Good food is homemade from farm-fresh ingredients. Preferably by someone who is a great cook and loves us a lot; those are all the ingredients we need. So let me ask, do you cook? Do your kids know how to cook? When was the last time you made a meal? What is more important than creating a meal for your family?

We have the most amazing abundance of fresh fruits and vegetables and meats and beautiful whole grain breads in our grocery stores and markets. But look in the shopping carts, what do most people buy? Boxes of food someone else cooked and chips, sodas, cookies, and ice cream. You need to cook for a lot of reasons. It's creative and fun and satisfying. It saves you money. Most important, it saves your health.

The freshest ingredients come from your garden. (Next best is from the farmer's market, the produce section in the grocery store, and then the freezer case.) Gardening is one of the best physical activities for you, too. Women who gardened for at least an hour a week in a research study had stronger bones than women who jogged. Sounds like several kinds of magic happen in the garden. If you have even the tiniest bit of earth, a deck, or windowsill where you can grow plants, or a community garden you can join, you can improve your health and your mealtimes—and give your kids the gift of learning to grow their meals.

Some schools have gardens where students grow their own food. Not surprisingly, these schools have the best lunch programs, too. Growing your own food is a valuable skill that no amount of technology can do better than you can. Does anything taste better than a homegrown tomato fresh off the vine? Would you even know?

Sensible Eating

If you're chewing something right now, don't take another bite. When you're driving, working, talking on the phone, or watching TV, you do not chew well, savor, or even taste what you are eating. That's not good. Food comes to you with a gift in its hands. Honor the miracle that food brings to you, and pay attention when you are eating.

You can't eat what isn't available. Bring home fruit and vegetables and whole grain crunchies; leave the Twinkies and chips back at the store. Then when you're hungry, your choices are all good!

Emotions can distract you from what you're eating, too. If you're angry—and please don't use dinnertime for yelling at each other or criticizing a family member—or you are sad or exhausted, you don't need food. You need a walk or a talk or a nap, but you don't need food just then.

If you're always going back for seconds, wait 15 minutes before you have a second helping. Chew thoroughly and slowly. Enjoy the quality of your food, not the quantity.

Be prepared for the times you always eat too much, such as church suppers, family reunions, and pot-luck meals after choir practice or high school football games. The cooks pull out all the stops to make the best dishes they can, and your taste buds go crazy. Eat less this time than you did at the last church supper. Eat foods, like vegetables, that have fewer calories than the desserts or fried chicken. Get up between servings and go thank the cooks.

Timing Is Everything

Do you eat more in the evening than any other time? If you want to lose some weight or not put on any more weight, shift your meals to different times. Stop saving your biggest meal of the day for last. Eat breakfast like a king. Once you stop eating so much in the evening, you will be hungry in the morning—I guarantee it. Have a good lunch, not just a bagel at your desk—and definitely don't skip it all together. You arrive home in the evening *starving* because you didn't eat during the day. This sets you up to eat for the next three or four hours.

If you have breakfast with protein and fiber in it, you feel full longer. A good lunch, and an afternoon snack of a piece of fruit and a handful of nuts, and you are fine with a smaller dinner, because you are not starving. Think about it. You are used to coming home and eating everything in sight, so go slow as you change this habit. Taking a walk in the evening before or after dinner can help change this habit to a healthier one. Eat slowly. Don't watch TV while you eat. If you want a bedtime snack, try popcorn or something with fiber that takes a while to eat and makes you feel full.

A Sheet of Paper with Writing on It

By the way, the only way you are ever going to know what you eat is to write it down. Keep a record for a couple of days. Some people start cutting back on things they usually eat because they have to write it down. Don't change anything yet. Write down *how much* you eat, too. A two-inch slice of sweet potato pie is different from half the pie. Serving size counts—maybe more than you know. If you want to lose a bit of weight but you don't want to change the foods you're eating, try smaller servings.

Don't starve yourself—don't ever do that—but be aware of what you are eating and spread your meals out over the day. It's best not to eat a huge meal at any time, but especially not in the evening when you can't burn that fuel before you go to bed.

The Building Blocks: Protein, Carbohydrate, and Fat

Okay, now it's time for the nuts and bolts of good eating. To be healthy, your body needs the basics—protein, carbohydrate, fat, vitamins, minerals, fiber, and water—and it needs them in the right amounts. Before long, you'll see that how much of something you eat can sometimes be more important than what you're actually eating. But let's start from the beginning and talk about what's in the food we eat and why we need to it.

Rising Stars—Protein and Carbohydrate

You may have heard a lot about carbohydrate (carb) and protein recently. A lot of new diets have focused on these two nutrients and the role they play in weight gain. So where do you find carb and protein?

Protein is found in:

- Meats—beef, pork, chicken, turkey, fish

- Eggs

- Cheese and dairy products

- Nuts

- Beans

- Soy products like tofu

- Vegetables

Your body uses protein to grow and to make repairs. You don't need a lot of protein. If you limit foods with protein to one-quarter of your dinner plate or about as much as will fit in the palm of your hand, that's about right. Protein-rich foods shouldn't be the main attraction in your dinner, but it plays an important role. More than likely, you're getting more than enough protein to meet your daily needs. Most Americans get twice the protein they need in a day.

Carbs are found in:

- Grains—rice, noodles, grits, and cereals

- Breads—cornbread and biscuits

- Starchy vegetables—potatoes, peas, and corn

- Beans—limas, navy, pinto, kidney

- Milk—yogurt, ice cream

- Fruit

Carbohydrates are your body's favorite fuel. They make up most of the glucose your body uses for energy (we'll talk more about this later). The first four carb-heavy foods in this list should take up the same amount of space on your dinner plate as protein—about one-quarter. The last two carbs—milk and fruit—shouldn't really go on your plate, but they round out the meal. You can drink an eight-ounce glass of milk or eat a six-ounce cup of yogurt or pudding or ice cream. Fruit, such as an apple or a peach, is a perfect dessert.

Other vegetables, such as spinach and peppers, have carbs, but not so many as the starchy vegetables and other foods in the list above. Because vegetables have so many vitamins, minerals, and fiber, it's okay to eat huge servings— fill up half your plate with them. Have seconds!

Good Carbs, Occasional Carbs

Like fats, which we'll talk about shortly, not all carbs are the same. Some carb foods are better for you than others. Whole grains, fruits, and vegetables are powerhouses of vitamins, minerals, and fiber. Packed with all of these extra nutrients, these are the "good" carbs.

You also get carbs in desserts, cookies, crackers, snacks, and sodas—mostly from the sugar or white flour. When you

---

All These Carbs: What Can You Do?

- Drink water and ignore sugary drinks (other than milk).
- Bring home a variety of fruits and vegetables. Eat them.
- Cut down on the cookies, chips, and snack foods. Save these for special occasions.
- Try fruit for snacks and dessert.
- Switch from regular soda to diet. Save soda for after your daily walk.
- Try snacks with fiber such as popcorn, whole grain crackers, or bean burritos.

---

eat these foods, you get a lot of calories but not many vitamins, minerals, or fiber. These are the "occasional" carbs. They are quickly digested, so your blood glucose spikes and then drops just as quickly. Soon your energy level plummets and you feel hungry again. Foods with fiber in them, like the good carbs, are digested more slowly and help you feel full and satisfied longer.

Try to keep a balance between good carbs and occasional carbs in your meals. Just because a food is an occasional carb, doesn't mean you have to completely cut it out of your diet. It's occasional, remember; you just need to compensate somewhere. You might skip the bread or rice at dinner if you want to have some cookies or a piece of pie for dessert.

Fats: What's Bread without Butter or Salad without Dressing?

Fats are perhaps the most infamous of our three nutrient building blocks. Over the past few decades fats have been demonized (a little unfairly), and most people believe that you shouldn't eat any fat at all. Fortunately, this isn't the case. You should definitely watch how much fat you're taking in, but fats are still an important part of a balanced diet.

Fats are found in:

Bad	Good
Butter	Vegetable oils
Lard	Nuts
Margarine	Seeds
Meats	Olives
Milk, cheese, yogurt	Avocados

Fats taste good and help us feel full. But just like carbs, it is important to know that there are "bad" fats and "good" fats.

Bad fats are called saturated fats. They come mainly from animals—think hamburger. They are in the list on the left with butter and cheese. These fats are solid at room tempera-ture, like bacon grease. The saturated fat in these bad fatty foods is the kind that clogs up your arteries (especially if you don't get any exercise) and is hard on your heart.

A healthy step you can take is to cut down on the amount of red meat (hamburgers, steak, and ribs) and whole and 2% milk (cheese, butter, and ice cream) you and your children eat. Try lean meats, such as chicken, turkey, or fish. Try vege-tarian dishes, such as bean burritos or vegetable stir-fry. Try low-fat cheese. If you're feeling adventurous try soy prod-ucts, such as textured soy protein, which looks and tastes like meat in chili and stews but doesn't give you saturated fat.

The good fats are unsaturated fats. They come from plants and are liquid at room temperature—think olive oil and canola oil. These fats are in the list on the right. They are important to every cell in your body. They help keep your heart healthy and your blood vessels flexible. In fact, research shows that if you eat a handful or two of almonds every day, the good fats and vitamins in almonds lower cholesterol levels and benefit your heart. Your fat choices should be from the good list. Cut back on fats from the bad list. Sprinkle nuts or sesame seeds on your salad or stir-fry vegetables in olive oil.

Figure 2-1. Ingredients List

> **INGREDIENTS:** ENRICHED PASTA, PARTIALLY HYDROGENATED VEGETABLE OIL, BROCCOLI, WHEY MALTODEXTRIN, CHEDDAR CHEESE (PASTEURIZED MILK, CHEESE CULTURES, SALT, ENZYMES, BUTTERMILK)

What about Margarine?

You may have noticed that margarine was sitting on the bad-fat side of the list above. Yes, it is made of vegetable oil, which is a good fat, but the vegetable oil has been treated with hydrogen to make it hard. Hydrogenated vegetable oil is a saturated fat, also called trans fat. Trans fats show up in fried fast foods, such as French fries and fried chicken. Trans fats are also in most packaged crackers, cookies, and baked goods. Soon, all product manufacturers will have to list trans fat on the Nutrition Facts label printed on food packages. Until then, you can find out if a product has trans fats in it by checking the list of ingredients for hydrogenated vegetable oil (see Figure 2-1).

Trans fats are about the worst fat there is. You want to cut down on trans fats. Since they hide in packaged snacks and desserts and fried fast foods, leave them behind at the store. Buy margarine that is not made from trans fat (check the ingredients label). Making your own cookies with whole-wheat pastry flour can be a healthier choice, and it's more fun than just buying a package of cookies. It's an activity you can share with your children.

The Protein and Fat Combo

The beef in a burger is red meat protein. It comes with saturated fat. A soy burger, on the other hand, has plant protein

One Change Changes It All
If you want to make just one healthy change to your meals, add three vegetables (that aren't potatoes!) and two pieces of fruit every day. That's 5-a-day. If you want to be beautiful, smart, AND sexy, eat more fruits and vegetables!

and even with cheddar cheese on top, it has less saturated fat than a regular burger. If you're not quite ready for soy, try ground turkey or chicken. These are lean meats that have less saturated fat than beef—especially when the skin has been removed. Fish is lean protein low in saturated fat. Nuts and seeds have plant protein and good unsaturated fat.

It is wise to eat a variety of protein foods. If you or your children always eat a cheeseburger and fries for lunch or dinner, you are getting too much red meat, too much milk protein, and too much saturated fat to be as healthy as you want to be. Try to get your protein from more chicken, fish, turkey, beans, and skim milk products.

Vegetables of Many Colors

Fresh fruits and vegetables—five of them every day—may be the most important key to good health. They have vitamins and minerals and lots of different colors and tastes to keep you from getting bored. Do you eat vegetables every day? Look at your dinner plate. What colors are there? Brown meat, brown potatoes, brown gravy, yellow corn, white bread?

Get some green and red and orange on that plate. Have a salad of mixed field greens, romaine or spinach, and tomatoes. Try collards, kale, or wilted spinach and onions. Eat okra and squash and peppers of all colors. Add oranges to your plate with carrots, sweet potatoes, pumpkin, and squash.

The Kids Don't Like Vegetables?

Most kids like potatoes and maybe corn, so that's what their parents serve. Potatoes and corn are protein and starch. Introduce your children to the wider world of vegetables. Most kids quickly learn to like broccoli and sweet potatoes and raw veggies like cucumber, carrots, and red peppers. But a new vegetable has to show up on the plate about 10 times before the child even knows how it tastes. Keep trying, and they'll come around. And be sure to eat your vegetables, too. Be proud of how wise your family is becoming.

There is a great website—*www.Kidnetic.com*—that can help make good nutrition and exercise fun for you and your kids. It is sponsored by five organizations: the American Academy of Family Physicians, American College of Sports Medicine, American Dietetic Association, International Life Sciences Institute Center for Health Promotion, and the National Recreation and Park Association. There are no food commercials to interrupt the video fun and games. It's got some great games and some great recipes for different categories, such as Gross Out Delights and Brown Bag Specials. There's also a section on fun and games the family can do together.

5-a-Day

When you build your meals around five vegetables and fruits a day, you take a giant step forward. And it's easier than counting calories. When you've become a master at fruits and vegetables, you may want to graduate to the National Cancer

Tip
If your family loves barbecue, but doesn't love vegetables, how about barbecuing the vegetables?

Institute's goal of nine servings of fruits and vegetables a day. Yes, they are that important. Just remember, an apple (or five) a day keeps the doctor away.

What Is So Special about Fiber?

Fiber is the part of a plant that cannot be digested. It makes you feel full. If you have diabetes, it helps keep your blood sugar on an even keel. It even helps lower cholesterol levels. It keeps everything moving smoothly through your digestive tract and prevents constipation. You find fiber in fruit, vegetables, whole grains, beans, and peas. On a food label in the Nutrition Facts, fiber is listed under Total Carbohydrate (see Figure 2-2).

Researchers have found a connection between eating lots of fiber and a decrease in the growths called polyps that often lead to colon cancer. You want to eat 20 to 30 grams of fiber a day. The average American eats only about 10 grams of fiber a day. Look for foods that add fiber to your meal. You don't have to eat bran flakes every morning—you'll be surprised what foods have fiber in them. Try apples, beans, berries, broccoli, brown rice, carrots, grapes, pears, peas, peppers, oatmeal, and shredded wheat. Look at the food label!

Fiber is one of the reasons why a cup of beans is better for you than a cup of white rice. White flour, white rice, and grits have had the fiber removed. If you want grits for breakfast, add 1/2 cup of wheat bran and 1 Tablespoon of water while they're cooking. This won't change the taste, and it replaces the fiber. The next time you choose bread, cereal, or grain, go for the rich color and power of whole grains.

What's Wrong with Sugary Drinks?

The simple fact is that too many people in the United States drink too much soda. They drink it for breakfast, lunch, din-

Figure 2-2. Nutrition Facts Label

Nutrition Facts

Serving Size 1 cup (228g)

Servings Per Container 2

Amount Per Serving

Calories 260 Calories from Fat 120

	% Daily Value*
Total Fat 13g	**20%**
Saturated Fat 5g	**25%**
Cholesterol 30mg	**10%**
Sodium 660mg	**28%**
Total Carbohydrate 31g	**10%**
Dietary Fiber 0g	**0%**
Sugars 5g	
Protein 5g	

Vitamin A 4%	•	Vitamin C 2%
Calcium 15%	•	Iron 4%

* Percent Daily Values are based on a 2,000 calorie diet. Your daily values may be higher or lower depending on your calorie needs:

	Calories:	2,000	2,500
Total Fat	Less than	65g	80g
Sat Fat	Less than	20g	25g
Cholesterol	Less than	300mg	300mg
Sodium	Less than	2,400mg	2,400mg
Total Carbohydrate		300g	375g
Dietary Fiber		25g	30g

Calories per gram:

Fat 9 • Carbohydrate 4 • Protein 4

ner, snack time—pretty much all the time. A 12-ounce can of regular soda has 10 to 14 teaspoons of sugar in it and 150–200 calories. At each meal, you could be gulping 20 spoonfuls of sugar and 250 calories on top of the food you're eating. This may be the "food" that is causing you and

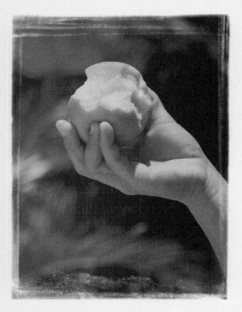

your children to weigh too much. We were not made to drink so many calories. It's better to chew them.

What can you do about it? You can change to diet soda, but be careful. Too much artificial sweetener can cause nausea and diarrhea. Drink more water instead. Try water with meals and save the soda for a reward after your daily walk. Think about when and why you drink soda, and see what small changes might work for you, because this first small change is the most important change to make.

If you don't drink sodas, but choose fruit juice or sports beverages like Gatorade, take a look at what you're drinking. Fruit juice and sports beverages are sugary drinks, too, even if they are healthier than soda. And most people don't drink just a tiny glass of juice—it's usually huge. Still, real fruit juice (not Hawaiian Punch or Gatorade) does have a lot of nutrients your body needs, so go ahead and have a glass, just make sure it's in the little glass.

Milk has natural sugar, too. It is one of the healthier choices of sugary beverages that provide us with carbohydrate. It's also one of the best sources of calcium there is. If milk doesn't agree with you—if you are lactose intolerant—you might try lactose-free milk, soy milk, or lactase enzyme pills that you take with regular dairy products.

Tea Is More than Tasty

In almost every single country other than the United States, tea is the drink of choice. For some reason, it just hasn't

---

Drink More Water

Get a pitcher or jug of water and fill it up in the morning. You can see how much water you drink during the day. Aim for 6 to 8 glasses full. Sodas don't count, but tea does.

---

caught on here. But that is changing, and for good reason. You might want to consider drinking more tea, because it contains strong disease fighters. Research done at the Antioxidants Research Lab at Tufts University in Boston shows that tea—whether it's green, black, red, or white—has health benefits. Tea contains antioxidants that protect you against heart disease and some forms of cancer. Some people prefer herbal tea and avoid regular tea because of the caffeine, but herbal teas do not have the same antioxidant power. If you're worried about the caffeine, you could choose red tea, also called rooibos (roy-boss) tea from South Africa. It has no caffeine but does have high levels of antioxidants. Research shows that your heart gets benefits from two cups of tea a day, but drinking four or five cups spread out over the day, as folks do in China and Japan, is even better.

Unsweetened bottled tea is a better choice than soda (check the label to make sure it's unsweetened), but it only has about half the antioxidants of freshly brewed tea. Making your own is cheaper and better for you. A pound of tea can make 300 cups of tea. A pound of coffee can make about 40 cups of coffee. Tea is a bargain drink!

In the South, we like sweet tea, with 3 or 4 teaspoons of sugar in every glass. If you usually order presweetened tea, ask for unsweetened tea and just use a teaspoon of sugar. This is a small change you soon get used to.

Alcohol

Studies show that one small drink containing alcohol a day, such as a glass of wine with dinner, may improve your heart health. If you don't drink, this is no reason to start, but if you enjoy a glass of wine or beer and your doctor says it's okay, go ahead. It raises your HDL (good) cholesterol level, but if your triglyceride level is above 500, alcohol will make it worse. Also, if you have more than 3 drinks, alcohol raises your blood pressure. We know that more than 3 drinks may mean other problems, too.

How Much Is Enough?

A lot of folks don't realize that how much you eat is just as important as what you eat. A half cup of ice cream could fit into anyone's daily meal plan. A pint couldn't. It's not the ice cream that is bad; it's how much of it you're eating.

Unfortunately, most people do not know what size a serving size is. What the heck does a 3-ounce piece of meat look like? If the recipe says it makes 6 servings and each serving is one cup, you may need to measure. At our house when I was young, a cup could be a couple of different sizes. When it was something good, I wanted my daddy's cup. When it was something bad, I wanted my momma's cup. I'm sure you can guess which was the big one and which was the small one. Servings of carb foods like rice and pasta belong in momma's cup. Servings of vegetables belong in daddy's cup. Better yet, use a real measuring cup!

Look at your dinner plate. Is it about 10 inches across? You really don't need a plate bigger than that. In fact, some people find an easy way to cut back on the amount of food they eat is just to use smaller plates and bowls. It's a trick of the eye, but it works. If you're the kind of person who always cleans their plate, try cleaning a smaller one.

The Plate Method

Now keep looking at your plate. Draw an imaginary line and cut the plate in half and then in half again so there are four sections. This makes an X on the plate. One section is for meat or another protein-heavy food. One section is for starch or carbs, such as rice, pasta, or potatoes. The other two sections are for vegetables. You can pile the veggies pretty high, unless of course, they're fried. So no, those French fries don't count. They go in the starchy-carb quarter of the plate.

The Incredible Giant Serving

People may eat too much because they are given too much food. Restaurant serving sizes have really grown over the past 20 years.

Let's start with the drinks. A normal sized Coke used to be an eight-ounce glass bottle. Today Coke comes in 20-ounce plastic bottles and one person drinks the whole thing. That bottle contains 70 grams of carbohydrate, 14 teaspoons of sugar, and 250 calories. Did you know that? You'd

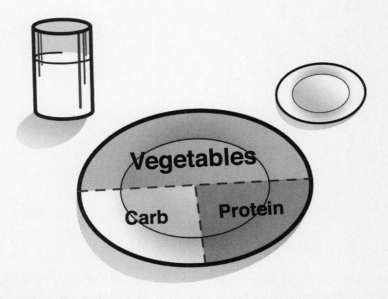

Crunching the Calories

If you're trying to eat 2,000 calories a day, where do foods like these fit?

Large French fries	600 calories
Cheese fries	3,000 calories
Carrot cheesecake (small slice)	1,560 calories
Denny's French toast	1,000 calories

When you walk one mile you burn 100 calories.
One plate of cheese fries = thirty miles.
That's a lot of walking for an appetizer.

have to eat 7 cups of broccoli to get the same amount of carbs. If you have diabetes, the liquid carbs send your blood sugar through the roof. You have to chew broccoli, which slows down the food being digested, and it has fiber in it, which slows digestion a bit more.

A serving of French fries used to have 210 calories, and a lot less French fries. Now it's super sized and comes with a whopping 600 calories. When you eat this serving, you have enough fuel to walk for 2 hours!

Most dinners at chain family restaurants, which are often heavily fried, are served in four serving helpings. If you eat just half the food on the plate you're eating more than your body was designed to take in.

You can make a difference in your weight and your health by skipping the soda and stopping before you take the last three bites of your hamburger. Or by walking an extra mile today. Or by a combination of the two. Little changes add up to a lot over time.

Know Your Delicious Fishes

The American Heart Association recommends we eat fish twice a week for the heart-healthy omega-3 fats. As you do with your choices of vegetables and fruits, eat a variety of fish, not just one kind.

Our oceans and rivers and plants that grow in them have become contaminated with mercury, a metal that is toxic to humans. Little fish eat the plants and the mercury too. Big fish, like tuna, eat a lot of little fish and may have quite a bit of mercury in them. If you eat fish like tuna three times a week, you may get too much mercury in your body. It can affect the nervous system and cause symptoms such as dizziness, memory loss, numbness, and hair loss. If you stop eating that type of fish for a few weeks or eat other types of fish, your body will get rid of the mercury in a short time. Look at Table 2-1. One Fish, Two Fish to see which types of fish tend to have the most mercury.

The danger is for unborn babies and growing children, because mercury can cause permanent damage to their developing brains and nervous systems. That's why pregnant women and children should not eat fish that may have high levels of mercury in them.

Farm raised fish have less mercury than ocean fish and certain types of fish generally have more mercury than others. For example, salmon gives you high levels of healthy omega-3 fats, with little mercury.

Beware of the Low-Fat Diet

Some people think that a low-fat diet is the way to lose weight. It may be, but some types of fat are important to your daily health. We need about 10 to 15% of our food to be in the form fats, fats that our body can't make. These are called essential fatty acids. Make sure that you get enough good, unsaturated fat every day.

Table 2-1.   One Fish, Two Fish

OK anytime	Mercury Levels	Omega-3 Levels
Catfish	low	low
Clams	low	low
Orange Roughy	low	low
Oysters (Pacific)	low	high
Oysters (Elsewhere)	low	medium
Salmon	low	high
Sardines	low	high
Shrimp	low	low
Tilapia	low	low
OK some of the time	**Mercury Levels**	**Omega-3 Levels**
Flounder	medium	medium
Mahimahi	medium	low
Red Snapper	medium	low
Trout	medium	high
Not OK	**Mercury Levels**	**Omega-3 Levels**
Amberjack	high	low
Chilean Sea Bass	high	medium
Grouper	high	low
Halibut	high	low
Shark	high	medium
Swordfish	high	medium
Tuna	high	high

Adapted from *Health* magazine, June 2003, p. 124.

Before you buy a "low-fat" food, please read the food label. Many low-fat foods have more sugar in them than the regular version to make up for the change in taste when the fat is removed. The result is less fat, but usually the same amount of calories. You may also notice that even low-fat foods have a serving size on the label. A lot of people think that just because a food is low-fat, they can eat the whole box.

Still, most people eat too much fat and need to cut down on how much they're taking in. Fat packs more calories per gram (nine calories to be exact) than carbohydrate and protein (which have four), so it just makes sense that if you want to drop pounds, you're going to want to drop fat. Fortunately, there are thousands of ways to trim fat from your diet without having to sacrifice too much taste. For example, if you're like me, you can't give up having gravy every day. But gravy is made from pan drippings and milk, which have saturated fat. How about using one tablespoon of pan drippings with some canola oil or light olive oil and stirring in low-fat or nonfat milk? You could try whole-wheat pastry flour instead of white flour to thicken it. Or you could just put regular gravy on top of brown rice and vegetables. You have choices!

Ways to Cut the Fat When You Cook

- Use olive oil or canola oil instead of lard, butter, or margarine.
- Use a nonstick cooking spray for sautéing or pan-frying.
- Add small amounts of nuts, nut butter, seeds, or avocado instead of butter or margarine.
- Try canola, soy, or reduced-fat mayonnaise, or make your own by mixing equal parts of mayonnaise with one of the following:
  - Mustard
  - Skim or low-fat milk
  - Plain low-fat or nonfat yogurt
  - Fat-free sour cream
  - Blended tofu
- Cook turkey or chicken with the skin on but remove it before eating.
- Cook meat on a rack so the fat drips off. George Foreman has a good grill for this.
- Baste with juice, wine, or broth instead of butter or meat fat.
- Cook soups and stews ahead of time and refrigerate. The fat will rise to the top and harden, so you can remove it. Or you can use an ice cube wrapped in a paper towel to skim fat from the hot soup.

(Continued)

Ways to Cut the Fat When You Cook (*continued*)

- Replace part of the meat in a recipe with beans, vegetables, or grains.

In fried foods:

- Use a well-seasoned iron skillet or other high-quality pan.
- Heat the pan before adding oil—this prevents food from sticking.
- Use only fresh oil—never reheat oil and use again.
- Heat the oil until it is hot but not smoking. If the oil is not hot enough, the food will absorb too much of it and taste greasy.
- Watch the pan closely and remove food quickly when done, and drain it on several paper towels.
- Serve light dishes for the rest of the meal: low-calorie vegetables, salad, and fruit for dessert.

Instead of:	Try:
Bacon slices	Soy bits (bacon-flavored) or 1 Tbsp finely chopped bacon
Bacon fat, shortening, lard, butter, or margarine	Olive oil, canola oil, peanut oil, nut butters
Cream	Evaporated skim milk, plain nonfat yogurt, blended tofu
Cheese	Reduced-fat cheeses
Salt, salty seasonings	Herbs, lemon, garlic, hot sauce
Regular bouillon and canned broth	Homemade stock, low-sodium broths, low-sodium bouillon powder
High-fat meat for seasoning (ham hocks, fatback, bacon)	Lean ham, turkey bacon, lean pork chops, turkey wing (skin off), leftover chicken

Adapted from *Southern Style Diabetic Cooking* by Marti Chitwood, RD, CDE, ADA. American Diabetes Association, 1996.

A Simple Meal Plan

Perhaps it will help you to see what a meal plan is. Then you can look at the food choices that you make every day in a new light. Eat breakfast. Most overweight people don't eat breakfast. You can breakfast like a king because you burn those calories throughout the rest of the day. Good choices are oatmeal, all-bran, or whole grain cereal with pecans and raisins and cinnamon, berries, peaches, or bananas. Choose a fruit you like. You might have scrambled eggs and toast. Or a whole grain muffin, egg, yogurt, and fruit. Or a milkshake made with yogurt and fresh fruit.

Use the food label to help you choose cereals. Is whole-wheat or another whole grain the first thing on the ingredients list? How much sugar is on the list? Check the Nutrition Facts. If the cereal has three or more grams of fiber, it's likely to be whole grain. Same goes for bread. These are good choices!

The following is a good, healthy, sensible meal plan for a day. It looks like a lot of food, doesn't it? That's because it is. But all of the food choices are good choices. How does this compare to your daily eating?

Breakfast: A bowl of oatmeal with pecans and cinnamon, milk, and a peach.

Snack: A piece of fruit and a slice of cheese or a handful of almonds.

Lunch: Lean meat or cheese sandwich, soup or salad, and a piece of fruit.

Snack: 1/2 lean meat or peanut butter sandwich on whole wheat bread, 1/2 cup carrot sticks.

Dinner: 1 large slice baked ham, 1 cup white beans, 1 piece corn bread with butter, 2 cups collard greens, 1/2 cup ice cream with 1 tablespoon chocolate syrup.

Snack: 3 cups popcorn and a glass of water.

A Diabetic Diet?

A lot of my patients who have diabetes ask me for a diabetic diet. You may be wondering the same thing. I'll tell you what I tell them: There is no such thing as a diabetic diet. As we say in church, let me repeat that: *There is no such thing as a diabetic diet.* Go and tell everyone I said so. Healthy foods are healthy for everyone, even folks with diabetes. A healthy diet is good for your heart, your brain, your blood vessels, your organs, your muscles, skin, and bones, too. The best idea is to start with the foods you're already eating every day. How healthy are they? And how much are you eating? Even healthy foods go wrong when you eat enough for five people. Many people make their first step to eat smaller servings.

Another misconception is that people with diabetes can't eat sugar. This is not true. Sugar is just another carbohydrate. As you know, it's not one of the good carbs, but you can fit it

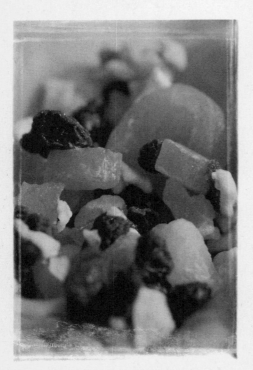

into a meal by trading other carbs for it. The important point is that carbohydrate raises your blood sugar, whether it's coming from a soda or a slice of bread. It helps to learn to count the amount of carbohydrate in each food. For example, a slice of bread, an apple, and a glass of milk all have about the same amount of carb—15 grams each. So breakfast with a piece of toast, a glass of milk, and an apple will have 3 × 15 grams of carb in it, or 45 grams of carb.

If you eat the same amount of carbohydrate at breakfast each day—different foods, but with the same amount of carb—then your blood sugar levels fall into a pattern you can predict. Same goes for the same amount of carb at lunch and dinner. You might aim for 60 grams of carb at breakfast, 75 at lunch, and 75 at dinner. You don't have to be exactly on the number, but keeping the carb count in the ballpark is good for your blood sugar. You should have an appointment with a registered dietitian, who can help you plan your meals with foods that you like. She'll help you learn carb counting and how to take good care of your diabetes.

The Mediterranean Diet and Preventing Disease

Maybe you're heard that eating like the French or the Greeks is a healthy way to eat. Maybe you've just heard the part about having a small glass of wine with dinner. But to get the benefits, you need to eat all the foods in their meals, especially the one pound of vegetables that they eat every day. And you need a stress-relieving daily walk to copy their more relaxed pace of life, too.

Anyway, they eat the same healthy foods that we have been talking about—vegetables, fruits, whole grains, fish, nuts, and olive oil. They do eat a lot of olive oil on all those vegetables, but these healthy oils are the only oils they get. They don't eat unhealthy fast food fats. The healthy fats they eat are very important to your health. In fact the Lyon Diet Heart Study in France found that people eating the Mediterranean way were healthier than people on the low-fat American Heart Association diet. Recent research shows that this way of eating (and walking) really cuts your risk of heart disease, cancer, and other things that cause people to die too young.

The Secrets of the Mediterranean Diet

- Eat more fruit, vegetables, and fish.

- Cut back on red meat.

- Use olive oil instead of butter and cream.

- Walk every day.

Spotlight on Healthy Restaurant Eating

There is no doubt about it; we eat out more often than ever before. Why is this a problem? Well, besides busting your wallet, it's busting your belly. Just one restaurant meal a week adds an extra 600 calories or more to your fuel tank. Every time you eat out, you'll need to walk two hours to burn up those extra calories. Can you keep up with the number of times you eat out?

Most moms now work outside the home, which translates into their families eating more fast food, take-out food, frozen dinners, and catch-as-catch-can dining because mom is tired and too busy to cook.

If you're going to eat out, you need some tools to do it wisely. Keep these things in mind while you've got a menu in your hand:

1. Ask for salad dressing and sauces on the side so you can put on a little instead of a lot. There's a lot of fat and calories hiding in these toppers.
2. Ask for meat or fish to be broiled or grilled instead of fried.
3. Look for dishes with more vegetables and less meat and cheese.
4. Ask for one whole-wheat roll instead of a whole loaf of garlic bread, please.
5. Drink water or unsweetened tea.

6. If the meal is large, ask for a take-home container, and divide it before you eat. Take the other half home and have it for lunch tomorrow.

7. Divide dessert with your family or friends. I have a friend who always claims, "I never eat dessert." His wife is quick to add, "No dear, you simply never *order* dessert." It's absolutely true. He always samples a little of everybody else's dessert instead. Maybe he's the one doing things right.

School Lunches and Our Children

Help your children prepare their own lunches. Even little kids can peel carrots, wash and tear lettuce, and make soup. And they are less likely to trade away something they helped choose and create.

Don't use food as a reward. You don't want your children to learn that food is a way to reward themselves for doing something good or to console themselves when they are sad or upset. Food is simply fuel for our bodies. Hugs and compliments are better to use for rewards and consolation.

If you can't control what they eat for lunch, make sure that their breakfasts and dinners are healthy. If they buy lunch at school, teach them the benefits of going for fewer burgers and more salads and soup. You can also talk to other parents about the lunch situation. Work together with the school to improve your children's school lunches.

Busy moms and everyone else need quick and easy recipes. You may have to go to the library and check out some cookbooks, buy a cooking magazine or cookbook, or check out some websites to find some new recipes that look interesting and healthy. You'll probably do better if you start making a shopping list, using the new recipes to decide what you need to buy. Cooking can be a lifelong hobby that brings you and your family joy as well as good health.

Toolkit for Eating Right
• Eat three vegetables and two fruits every day.
• Eat dinner earlier.
• Eat breakfast.
• Eat lunch.
• Eat a variety of foods, not the same two or three over and over.
• Try smaller meals.
• Trade tea or water for sweet beverages.
• Pack your lunch.
• Bring home good stuff to eat.

Resources

Online

For a fun place for kids to learn about food and nutrition visit:
www.KIDNETIC.com

For information about organic foods and their benefits:
www.theorganicreport.org

Associations

American Dietetic Association
216 West Jackson Boulevard
Chicago, IL 60606
800-877-1600
www.eatright.org

American Diabetes Association
1701 N. Beauregard St.
Alexandria, VA 22311
800-DIABETES
www.diabetes.org

International Food Information Council Foundation
1100 Connecticut Avenue, NW
Suite 430
Washington, DC 20036
202-296-6540
www.ific.org

This organization communicates science-based information on health, nutrition, and food safety. It is supported by food, beverage, and agricultural industries. Offers free brochures on nutrition and health.

3

BEING ACTIVE IS BEING ALIVE

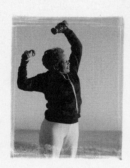

I'd do anything to look like all these beautiful people you see here tonight—except, of course, exercise and eat right!

—Steve Martin, 2003 Academy Awards

As you can see from the quote, the truth can be funny. We all know that exercise is good stuff and that it does wonderful things. So why don't any of us do it? To tell you the truth, I'm less concerned about fussing at people about their eating if they are really working at their exercise. Why not follow the example of the beautiful people and exercise? All your health problems will improve. Or you won't develop any. Every type of physical activity, from mountain climbing to sex, benefits your health. Just plain old walking, when you do it everyday, is exercise enough to get all these benefits. We have the research to prove it—exercise and food have a better effect on your health than any drug.

Is exercise worth it? Yes! Almost every aspect of your health is either maintained or improved by physical activity. The long list of beneficiaries from exercise includes:

- Your fat level
- Your muscles
- Your blood pressure
- Your cholesterol levels
- Your blood sugar levels
- Your bone density
- Your strength and balance
- Your appearance
- Your mood
- Your sleep
- Your quality (and quantity) of life

The biggest improvements from exercise show up in your circulatory system. Research shows that regular exercise reduces blood pressure by about 10 points on the top and bottom numbers. It makes your heart stronger. Exercise is also like a natural aspirin, relieving pain and helping to keep your blood flowing smoothly. Exercise can promote the growth of new blood vessels around small blockages in the blood vessels in your legs. It raises HDL (good) cholesterol, lowers total cholesterol, and decreases triglyceride levels for 48 hours afterward.

For people with diabetes, exercise lowers your A1C and your fasting glucose levels. This is because when you exercise your muscles take glucose directly from the bloodstream, without the need for insulin. You can use up to 20 times more glucose than usual. See for yourself. Check your blood sugar before you exercise and then 30 minutes afterward. It keeps lowering glucose for 24 hours afterward, too. Then, as you keep exercising and building muscle, your body will use glucose more and more efficiently.

Your immune system also benefits from regular physical activity. Exercise decreases the number of colds and respiratory infections you get. It also decreases your chances of serious diseases, too, like colon and breast cancer.

But perhaps most important, and most often overlooked, is that exercise relieves anxiety and is a good way to work through emotions. It releases feel-good brain chemicals, called endorphins, which are more powerful than morphine. If you're feeling stressed from all the chaos in your life, take a long walk or ride your bike or go for a jog. You'll find that after a half hour of good exercise, all those problems don't seem so big or so complicated. Hey, exercise is good stuff. I often remind my students and trainees that for all of the worst metabolic diseases affecting this nation's citizens, whether obesity, diabetes, or hypertension, the first treatment recommendation is the same—exercise and improved eating habits.

The Reasons We Don't Exercise

I'll wager that all of this information is not new to you. We all know we need to exercise. Still, most of us simply don't. Why? There are a million excuses, but the three reasons people most often give for not exercising are:

- Not enough time

- Pain or injury

- No place to do it.

Let's look at these excuses a little more closely.

Lack of Time

This one is very popular. Interestingly, though, most people still have enough time to watch an average of four hours of TV a day. Turn off the TV and get moving. Get your kids to go with you . . . in the stroller or a backpack, riding their bikes, or walking alongside you. Trade workout time with your spouse if one of you needs to watch the children or make dinner or do whatever the chore is. A daily walk is as important as the sleep you get every night and the food you eat every day. Just as important.

Pain or Injury

If you do have an injury, take care of it by staying off of it, massaging it, taking aspirin or whatever your doctor recommends. Then switch to another exercise that doesn't hurt the injury, such as swimming or riding a stationary bike. Be creative so you can keep getting the exercise that you need. Stretching and weights can be done sitting or lying down, so don't give them up if you don't have to. Hold the line.

No Place to Do It

Walk around your house. Dance around it. Walk around the block. If you only have a cul-de-sac, then walk around it. Join the walking group at the shopping mall. Get to work early and walk around the office floor. When your kids are at football or basketball practice, walk around the outside of the field. If you have a flight of stairs, put on some music and have fun climbing and descending to the different tempos. However you manage to do it, feel noble. Remember that you're setting an example for others, too. You're a great role model.

What about My Hair?

As Roniece Weaver, dietitian and author of the book *Slim Down Sister*, so wisely points out, black women who spend good money to get their hair looking beautiful on Saturday aren't going to want to sweat it out on Sunday afternoon.

Roniece's advice is to "get a weave." Since your health is the reason you are trying to be more active, please try to find a hairstyle that can hold up to exercise, so you will get out there and do it. She laughs when she says it, but she's as serious as I am about giving you the tools for good health.

Take the Time It Takes

A lot of people get discouraged with exercise very quickly. They think that if they don't drop twenty pounds in two weeks, then nothing is happening. Exercise won't change the appearance of your body immediately. The benefits on the inside start immediately, but it takes time to see them on the outside. Pilates claims you can see a difference in about a dozen sessions, but others take longer. What's a realistic goal for you? How about three months? If you don't even walk to the mailbox today, running a marathon within a month is not a very reasonable goal. Instead, try to be walking 3 miles a day within a year. Start by walking to the mailbox and back every day for several weeks. Then aim for the end of the block for a month or so. Then go all the way around the block, maybe for a month. As you get stronger, you can go farther. Give yourself time to enjoy it. While you walk, listen to books on tape, which you can check out from the library. Listening to a good murder mystery is a great to get your walking pace and your heart rate up. Some people who walk on treadmills like to treat themselves by watching their favorite TV program or video while they walk. Whatever you consider a treat, mix it with exercise, and you're more likely to keep exercising.

Keep in mind that exercise usually doesn't cause rapid weight loss. It's gradual, but if you stick with it, it's also certain. One or two pounds a week slip away. If you start the year out by walking to the mailbox, you may be walking three miles at a time at the end of the year. And losing

You're never too old to exercise
A lot of people complain that they've got too many years under their belt to start exercising. Well, I can tell you right now, you are never too old to exercise. Research in the frail elderly between 80 and 100 years old showed that they built muscle and strength lifting light weights. And not one of them had a heart attack or health problem brought on by exercise. If you have some health problems that you think might be a problem, talk to your doctor, who can give you a thorough physical and see what types of exercise would be good for someone in your position. There's always something you can be doing. As a wise person once said, you're never old enough to stop exercising.

62 pounds. Your friends who went with the three-week fad diet probably weigh more than they did when they started. The year is going to pass whether you sit it out or walk through it. Wouldn't you rather be sixty-some pounds lighter when it does pass?

Doctors and Exercise

Has a doctor ever told you that you need to get more exercise? Maybe not. Almost every study examining the factors that most improve health cites exercise as the number one positive influence on health, but most health care professionals don't talk seriously about it to people who aren't already doing it. It is the key to the kingdom. If your doctor wrote you a prescription for exercise, would you follow it?

Your Exercise Prescription

When you have strep throat and your doctor gives you a prescription for an antibiotic, you go to the pharmacy and have it filled. Why? Because it will help you get better, right? Well, in this case, exercise is the medicine that's going to help you get better, so I'm going to write you a prescription. (If you have any medical conditions that you think might make it dangerous for you to do these exercises, talk with your doctor. He may be able to "prescribe" a better plan.)

Here is my exercise prescription for you and your school-age children. Go and get it filled. You'll get better, I promise:

1. *30-minute brisk walk, 3 times a week (Monday, Wednesday, and Friday), preferably after lunch or dinner.*
2. *One 45-minute walk on the weekend (Saturday or Sunday).*
3. *Lift 2-pound weights for 10 minutes, 2 times a week (Tuesday and Thursday).*
4. *Stretch for 10 minutes, 2 to 3 times a week (Monday, Tuesday, and Thursday), after walking or weight lifting.*

You may try walking at different times of day to see whether you are an early morning walker or evening walker. It's usually easier to stretch in the afternoon and evening because your muscles are warm from being used through the day. Always warm-up your muscles before you exercise and cool them down afterward.

When you pin down the details of what exercise to do, when to do it, and for how long, you can see how and where it fits into your day. You can't just say, "I'm going to exercise more." That's too broad and ambiguous. You need a step-by-step plan. A sensible approach is to "start low, and go slow."

Exercise Stress Test

Before you begin any exercise regimen, you should probably talk with your doctor about an exercise stress test, especially if you have health conditions like high blood pressure, heart disease, or diabetes. An exercise stress test checks the stress on your heart during exercise. This will be a good gauge for the amount and type of exercise you can do without over-exerting or injuring yourself. If you have a heart condition you should stay away from intense aerobic or resistance exercises at first. As your health improves you'll be able to do more. However, no matter what your condition, there will be some sort of physical activity you can do. The one that works for most everybody is to simply . . .

Walk!

As you can probably tell by now, I really like walking as a way to get you off your seat and moving. It's low impact, free, requires no special equipment other than a good pair of shoes, and almost anyone in the world can do it. There's really no reasonable excuse not to walk.

Still, a lot of people don't get moving. They're waiting for some miracle in a pill to do everything for them. If you're one of these people, think about this: A large research study recently showed that lifestyle changes are better than pills for

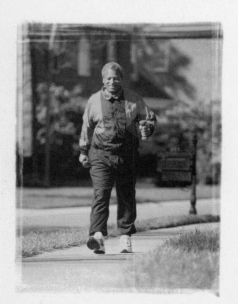

making you healthy. People in the study who walked 30 minutes a day cut their risk of developing type 2 diabetes by 30–40%. Yes, it's that simple. Do you have to walk every day? No, there are benefits no matter how many days you walk. But it's just common sense that the more days you walk, the more good you are doing for you.

People in the study who walked at least two hours a week—a 30-minute walk four

days a week, or an hour walk two times a week—cut their
risk of heart attack by more than one-third. But that's not all:
The people who walked briskly three to four hours a week
got the biggest health bonus of all. By walking 30 minutes
every day, they cut their chance of heart disease and diabetes
in half. Walking every day helps us humans live longer and
healthier lives. Don't you want a piece of this action?

Walking is different from pills in another important way.
It has no side effects. Well, that's not necessarily true. Maybe
we should say walking has side effects, it's just that they're
all good. Walking lowers body fat and cholesterol levels,
lowers blood sugar, and lowers your blood pressure. It would
take three or more different kinds of pills to try to copy those
results.

Keeping a Count—Pedometers

You probably have no idea how much walking you do in a
day. The best way to find out is to get a simple step counter,
or pedometer, that clips on your waistband. Wear it morning
to evening for several days to see how much walking you do.
The weekends may be more active for you, so include one of
those days, too. People who stay home all day generally don't
walk more than 2,000 steps a day. People who go out to
school or to work take about 4,000 to 5,000 steps a day. The
goal that is recommended for everyone—based on a lot of
research—is 10,000 steps a day. If you only walk 1,500 steps
now, your daily goal should be 1,700 steps for the next
two weeks. The next two to three weeks you can try for
1,900 steps a day. Start low, go slow. You can get to 10,000
steps a day if you build up to it.

Some pedometers measure every movement you make, so
you might pick up "steps" for just swiveling back and forth in
your chair at work. All movement is good, but you want to
take more actual steps in a day. Some pedometers, like the

Small Steps pedometer (mentioned below), filter out the jiggling. In fact, it doesn't record the steps until you have taken 5 of them.

Pedometers are fun for both kids and adults to wear, and they motivate you. When you can see that you only need 200 more steps for your daily goal, you're likely to take a quick 5-minute walk to push your total over the top. You can take about 100 steps in a minute and 1,000 steps in 10 minutes. Small walking breaks add up! Don't keep looking at the long-range goal. Just make a daily commitment to yourself. If you give yourself 3 or 4 hours a day to watch TV, you should have 30 minutes to take a walk and do something wonderful for yourself.

Small Steps Press, the publisher of this book, offers a pedometer and a 64-page Fast Facts walking book for $19.95. These products are available on-line at *http://store.diabetes.org* or by calling 1-800-232-6744. You can also find them at your local bookstore.

Variety Is Still the Spice of Life

I like walking, but it can't do everything. You need a well-rounded exercise program to get a lean, fit body. Besides, if you always do the same thing, you'll be as bored as your muscles are. Bicycling, skating, cross country skiing, swimming, golf, bowling, hop scotch, jumping rope—there are literally thousands of things you can do. Bring out the kid in you and have some fun.

There are several types of exercise and they each benefit your body. Of these types, there are three major varieties:

1. Aerobic exercise, such as walking or swimming, which works your heart and lungs.
2. Flexibility exercise, such as stretching or yoga, which stretches and strengthens muscles and improves your range of motion and balance.

Warm Up

Before starting any physical activity, you need to warm up
your muscles so you don't cramp or injure yourself. Start
by walking around for a few minutes. Stand with your arms
out at shoulder height and swing them around you in a
circle—25 times or so. Then stretch, like a cat waking up.
Reach up above your head with each hand, stretching from
toe to fingertip on each side. Arch your back and flatten it.
Put your hands against a wall or tree and lean forward to
stretch the tendons in the back of your legs and ankles.
Don't bounce; just hold it. There are some wonderful books
on stretching that you can check out of the library to learn
more stretches you may want to try.

---

3. Resistance or isometric exercise, which works your
    muscles against resistance, such as weights, to make
    them stronger.

Whatever exercise you choose to do, do it at a speed that
raises your heart rate but doesn't leave you so breathless you
can't talk. If you're breathless or your heart is pounding,
that's too fast. You want a moderate speed, so you can keep
going and going and going. Remember my rule: start low, go
slow.

Resistance Exercise Is Important

A lot of my patients feel that aerobic exercise and a little
stretching every now and then is all the exercise they need.
They say they don't want to be all muscled up and lumpy, so
why should they spend all that time lifting weights. I tell
them there are lots of reasons.

Physically and emotionally, working against resistance
makes us stronger. When you lift weights, the weight resists

your muscle from moving it. Your muscle has to work to move the weight. Your muscle gets stronger—strong enough to open jars and big heavy doors, to carry chairs, and to play with your children. Muscle keeps you independent all the way through old age. Muscle burns calories even at rest. Muscles are your friends.

Do you need to buy barbells? No. I always say that a 2-pound bag of rice weighs, what, nearly about two pounds? Find ways of doing things that work for you, that are possible for you. I've had patients use old retired pantyhose—whatever that means—to fill with sand to make a nice weight bag that you can grip easily. You can use them for resistance training, and you don't have to go buy weights. Cans aren't as easy to hold, but they do weigh something and since the weight is written on them, you know how much you're lifting. Bottles of laundry detergent have handles that might be easier for you to hold. Use your imagination to help yourself. Ask your doctor, nurse educators, and friends for ideas, too. Being creative and resourceful is another way to take control of your life.

Getting Started

Hopefully by now you have some ideas on ways to exercise. All you need to start is determination. Set a goal. Break the goal into four steps that you can take to reach it. Make a plan. Be patient. Don't try to be perfect. Don't get discouraged every time you slip up. Just make your goal realistic and stick with it and you can change your life. You pass on your values and beliefs to your children by your behavior . . . whether or not it's healthy behavior is up to you.

Rewards Are Important, Whether You See Them or Not

Reward yourself for exercising. Be proud of yourself and speak words of encouragement and love to your self. Enjoy

Table 3-1. Ways to Use Calories to Have Fun

How much you weigh, how fit you are, and how hard you exercise all have an effect on how many calories you burn, but this table can give you an idea of how many calories some physical activities burn based on your weight.

	Calories burned, by weight, after one hour		
	130 lb	155 lb	190 lb
Backpacking	413	493	604
Bicycling, leisurely	236	281	345
Bicycling, moderate effort, 12–14 mph	472	563	690
Canoeing and rowing, moderate effort	413	493	604
Dancing; jazz, ballet, modern, aerobic	354	422	518
Gardening, general	295	352	431
Golf, carrying clubs	325	387	474
Golf, pulling clubs	295	352	431
Golf, riding in a cart	207	246	302
Hiking, cross-country	354	422	518
Actively playing with children	236	281	345
Jumping rope, moderate	590	704	863
Softball or baseball	295	352	431
Swimming, leisurely	354	422	518
Tennis, singles	472	563	690
Volleyball, beach	472	563	690

Adapted from the "Activity List of NutriStrategy" (*www.nutristrategy.com/activitylist.htm*). These calculations are based on research data from *Medicine and Science in Sports and Exercise*, the official journal of the American College of Sports Medicine.

looking in the mirror! Enjoy feeling better, breathing better, sleeping better. Enjoy being able to climb the stairs to the third floor every day. Enjoy being able to keep up with your brother on a weekend run. These are all rewards in themselves. But sometimes you need to treat yourself for a job well done. Maybe you've earned some new clothes, too.

Do You Need to Sign a Contract?

You might be able to motivate yourself to exercise more often if you write out and sign a contract with yourself. This may work with children who believe in the power of giving their word. However, if you sign a contract with your child, please honor it. The child needs to see you keep your word to walk to better health alongside you. Signing an exercise contract usually has more meaning for adults who work in the business world or are retired from business and are used to signing contracts. It doesn't work so well for people who have never written or signed one.

Keeping a Journal

For some folks, writing in a journal helps them achieve goals and get things done that are important to them. The journal

---

Think About It

- What are your personal likes and dislikes when it comes to exercise?
- What forms of exercise do you like to do?
- Do you need help to learn about other kinds of exercise? Can you take a class, such as yoga or tai chi (Chinese gentle exercise with stretching and shifting-your-weight movements like a dance in slow motion)?
- You don't have to join a gym, but if you think you might exercise more there, go and see. Is it a welcoming place or a scary place?
- What do you like to wear when you exercise?
- Do you like to exercise with one other person, a group of people, or alone?
- Do you like to exercise outside or inside?
- Which family activities are actually active?
- Could you start an exercise group at church?

gives you information about yourself to work with. We know that very few people are truly aware of what and how much they eat—until they write it down. It's the same with exercise. It's your private journal, be honest. How else can you know where to start? People who use their journals for positive change and "hallelujah" results write down what they eat, what exercise they do, and what is going well or not going well in their daily lives. It helps to see on paper what you are doing now. This way you can figure out where you want to go.

When to Exercise?

Some people like to walk in the evening to wind down after a busy day. I know a lady who listens to books on tape as she walks around and around the block after dinner. The story on the tape is always different, so she doesn't mind covering the same ground. She feels that it's safe to walk in this neighborhood at night, too. If it weren't, she'd go over to the mall and walk inside.

Years ago, she and her young children, while they waited to join her husband in the military in Germany, had to move in with her parents. In part just to get out of the house, she started walking every morning at 6 A.M. She walked at least two hours, "to stay calm," she says with a smile. Since her parents were there with the kids, she didn't have to worry about them. She had been an aerobics instructor for a year so she didn't expect to see much change in her body, but after 4 months of daily long walks, her muscles were leaner

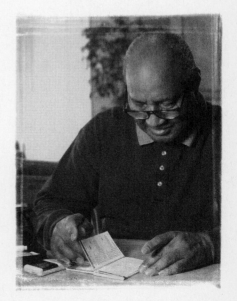

and longer. When she got to Germany, her husband declared that she had a new body.

It seems hard to believe that getting in shape is this simple. It is. Your challenge, of course, is to find the time to do it and then stay with it. If you work two jobs and you have little children, you are going to need some help. Or you are going to dance in the living room after they go to bed. Do whatever you can to get your daily physical joy.

Aisha Tyler, host of *Talk Soup* on E! and the character Charlie Weaver from NBC's *Friends,* told *SELF* magazine (Sept. 2003) that she prefers to do her yoga workout early in the morning. "If I don't exercise in the morning, I don't get it done. I feel invigorated and smile all day long. It makes me feel better about myself. I'm like, Whew! I just exercised! Did you?"

Magazines like *SELF* and *Men's Health* are good at giving you monthly doses of motivation and new ideas for being active. There is a *SELF* Challenge in March each year that lasts three months. During this period there are articles to help you focus on short-term goals, such as eating more greens during the week and stretching twice a week. *SELF* also provides a form each month for recording how you reached your goals for each type of exercise and healthy eating. Color photos and explanations help you achieve them. Women who try the challenge range in age from their teens to their 70s.

This year *SELF* added bonus points for various things, such as exercising with a friend or eating more than five vegetables in a day. You redeem bonus points when you can't do one of your workouts—or you just don't feel like doing it. This gives you a chance to rest or backslide or whatever you want to call it. Can you think of ways to award yourself bonus points so you don't feel so bad when you have to skip a walk or weights workout?

More Inexpensive Ways to Exercise

Walking isn't the only inexpensive form of exercise. You can find all sorts of ways to put steps into your day. Hide the remote control. Laugh—it burns calories and relieves stress. Walk the dog (who, as research on pets has shown, is also helping lower your blood pressure and stress levels). You can follow an exercise video or DVD. You can participate in an exercise class on TV. Look around, and you'll find lots of ways to be active.

Some churches already have Senior exercise classes. If yours doesn't, you might want to help get it started. It can be as simple as getting a bunch of friends together to go walking! The choir and the vestry can walk and talk instead of meet and eat.

Exercise Videos or DVDs

There are many exercise videos to choose from, so you can exercise at home on your schedule. There are videos for aerobic exercise to get your heart beating faster and your lungs working. There are videos for stretching, yoga, and Pilates. There are videos for lifting weights correctly, too. My wife and I have made great use of commercial exercise tapes over the years. Rent them from the video store or check them out from the local library to see how well they suit you before

More Fun Ways to Burn Calories		
Walking a dog	1/2 hour	100 calories
Shopping	2 hours	270 calories
Kissing	1 minute	1 calorie
Dancing	1 hour	350 calories

you buy them. There are programs to fit every need and style. My wife and I recommend alternating them to keep it interesting.

Now, some of you may feel uncomfortable about yoga, because you've heard that it is a religion. Yoga has different parts to it—spiritual guidance and physical exercise— because it is a way to live a long, healthy life. The focus of the "hatha" yoga that is primarily taught in the United States, however, is physical health. These stretches improve the strength, flexibility, and balance of your body. Yoga also teaches you to breathe more deeply, which is a great way to deal with stress and quiet your mind. This is exercise, not religion. But frankly, I'm hoping we all make exercise part of our religion.

Take a look at *Lilias Folan's Flowing Postures for Beginners* videos or her *Senior* series. She has been teaching yoga on television for more than 30 years, and she may be the perfect one to introduce you to the benefits of yoga.

TV Shows

There are exercise shows on TV, especially on PBS stations, covering everything from step aerobics to yoga and tai chi. Try one, try them all. It helps to have a variety of activities that you enjoy, so you don't get bored.

YMCA and City Recreation Departments

In most cities, local YMCA's and county recreation departments offer low cost exercise classes. Generally there are aerobics, jazzercize, stretching or yoga, tai chi, martial arts, and weight lifting. Many centers have indoor pools where you can join a water aerobics class or learn to swim if you don't know how. Check it out, there are as many classes for adults and senior citizens as there are for children. The whole family can enjoy and benefit from using the Y or the local recreation center. You could make your family's motto "Play more. Play harder. Have fun!"

Resources

Online

Operation FitKids (OFK) is the youth outreach program of the American College on Exercise. OFK provides schools with services to build a fitness program including equipment, educational materials, staff training, mentoring, and community partnering.
www.operationfitkids.com

The PBS website has an entire section devoted to personal health and wellness.
www.pbs.org/americaswalking/health

The President and the Department of Health and Human Services have created a health initiative for all Americans. To learn more visit:
www.healthierUS.gov

There you will also find links to a variety of government sponsored exercise and fitness programs, including:

- VERB: It's What You Do. This is a program to promote physical activity in young people.
  www.verbnow.com

- BAM: Body and Mind Kids Page.
  www.BAM.gov

The National Heart, Lung, and Blood Institute (NHLBI) and National Recreation and Park Association (NRPA) have worked together to develop Hearts 'N Parks, a program to help park and recreation agencies encourage heart-healthy lifestyles in communities. To learn more visit:

www.nhlbi.nih.gov/health/prof/heart/obesity/
hrt_n_pk/index.htm

Associations

President's Council on Physical Fitness and Sports
Department W
200 Independence Avenue, SW
Room 738-H
Washington, D.C. 20201-0004
202-690-9000
www.fitness.gov

American Council of Exercise (ACE)
4851 Paramount Drive
San Diego, California 92123
800-825-3636
www.acefitness.org

American College of Sports Medicine (ACSM)
P.O. Box 1440
Indianapolis, IN 46206-1440
317-637-9200
www.acsm.org

National Strength and Conditioning Association
4575 Galley Rd., Suite 400B
Colorado Springs, CO 80915
800-815-6826
www.nsca-lift.org

Books

Slim Down Sister, by Fabiola D. Gaines, RD, LD, and
Roniece Weaver, RD, LD, Angela Ebron. Plume, 2001.

Let's Get Real: Exercise Your Right to a Healthy Body, by
Donna Richardson, David Peden. Pocket Books, 1998.

The "I Hate to Exercise" Book for People with Diabetes, by Charlotte Hayes, MMSc, MS, RD, CDE. American Diabetes Association, 2001.

Small Steps, Big Rewards (walking book and pedometer). Small Steps Press, 2003.

The Healing Power of Exercise, by Linn Goldberg, MD, and Diane L. Elliot, MD. John Wiley & Sons, Inc., 2000.

Recorded Books Inc. produces lively audiobooks that are available at your local library or for rent or purchase by calling 1-800-636-3399 or online at *www.recordedbooks.com* and at local bookstores.

4

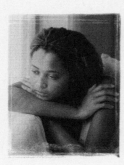

THE POWER OF EMOTION

I f you stay up to date with the latest advances in modern medicine, you will probably hear more and more about integrative medicine. This approach to healing considers the power of both the mind and the body. Your body has an immune system that is a marvel to behold in action. But the mind also plays an important role in helping to bring about healing. You and your physician should look at your mental and physical health and approach your healing through both doors. What you think and how you feel are important.

All this talk about illness and children suffering may scare you or depress you. It may make you mad. These are common emotions for people who are diagnosed with a chronic disease—or who have children with a chronic disease. It's human nature to feel that way.

Feel what you feel. Go ahead, cry, vent, get the sadness and anger moving on through.

Don't let them settle in. Suppressed or pent-up emotions affect our health through the stress they create inside us. Just getting mad at another driver on the way to work (which can often be an outlet for other frustrations in your life) creates enough stress in your body to elicit a physical response. We release five or more powerful hormones under stress, and hormones cause chemical changes in our bodies. For example, stress hormones raise both your blood pressure and your blood sugar.

I'm sure you've heard about the "fight or flight" hormones we release under stress, but nowadays, no one fights or runs away. We sit in traffic and quietly fume instead. Even if you do walk but you're worrying the whole time, you're under stress and making it harder for your body to be healthy. Pay attention to what you are thinking and how you are feeling. Feelings are not fixed and permanent. You can learn to let them flow over you and relax, even with stress in your life.

A New Viewpoint?

Some people might call anger or fear negative emotions, but they are useful. Anger is a way of saying, "Ouch, you stepped on my toe." It's simply feedback for those around you. It's only negative if you get stuck in that emotion or have truly unreasonable expectations of other people. Fear helps you focus in situations where you need to pay attention. But if you're afraid of everything, then fear is having a negative effect on your life.

Negative emotions aren't bad. They're part of life. You will have them. You can observe yourself having them. You can observe yourself behaving in certain ways because of the way you feel. And the minute you get enough distance from the feeling to watch yourself having it, you've got the power to move on.

Attitude Counts

The thing to remember about emotions is that you can make yourself feel so much worse than you already do. I know you're aware of this power. Watch how you talk to yourself inside your head. Watch how you talk about yourself to other people. Do you like you? Are you helping yourself by being encouraging and kind? Do you criticize yourself all the time? Whose voice is that? You have the power to turn off the voice that makes you feel bad and turn up the volume on the voice that is in love with you right now, the way you are now. Your closest companion is you. You might as well start liking yourself. How about seeing how much better you can make yourself feel right now? This is a critical element in taking control of your life.

If you deal with emotion like this—in a positive, self-reinforcing manner—you have created a whole new attitude and a different outlook on life. And you will need this change in your person. Why? When an illness is handed to you, you are being challenged to be stronger, calmer, wiser, and more spiritual than you've ever been. There is nobility in people facing a difficult challenge. Help yourself do it. Marshal your forces: get technical advice, get a support group, find out what you need to do, and do it. You always have the power to choose your attitude and your actions.

Our society goes to extraordinary lengths to avoid pain and to refuse to take responsibility for ourselves. The truth is that we have to be responsible for ourselves. Self-care is everything you do for yourself to remain healthy or to treat illness. You benefit from becoming part of the solution. Do your best and accept what happens. You will feel peaceful when you have done all you can.

Baby Steps Keep You from Tripping

Lifestyle changes are humbling because you have to start over. You have to learn new things, and you may be 65 and in no mood to start learning new things. Remaking yourself and restructuring lifelong habits can be daunting to a person who is comfortable with himself. You may be successful in business and very powerful, and you are not about to admit to any weakness. The truth is that we've all got challenges, so you're definitely not alone.

Look at the baby learning to walk. Does she sit there refusing to learn something new? No, she's driven by her curiosity and spirit to get up and keep trying, no matter how many times she falls down. Babies never quit until they succeed, even though it takes them months or years to conquer a new skill.

Learn from both her spirit and her method. She expects to fall down and doesn't waste energy fretting about that. She uses what she learns from each fall and stands up again. If you think of yourself as a toddler finding your way into a new world of experiences, it ought to make you smile. This is a hope-filled way to think of yourself. Laugh while you're learning. Meal planning, medicine regimens, exercise routines—all will be easier for you to learn, if you start with this attitude.

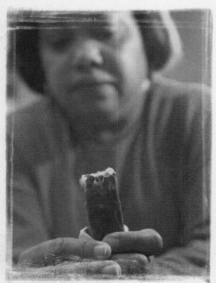

Making Changes

Before you can change, you have to have a good reason to change. But, this change should arise from a positive source, as a means to realize yourself more completely as a person. It should not be because you dislike yourself as you are. Think about it for a bit. What are the things that make you glad to get up in the morning? What do you enjoy doing or creating? What are your strengths? Make a list of all the things you do well. Then make a list of anything good that anyone has ever said about you. Positive things are more likely to encourage you to make changes in your life. Fear and negative thoughts don't motivate people to do much for long.

You set an example for others, whether you mean to or not. If you are cheerful, if you are coping with things that are hard for you, you are helping others cope, too. In return, you will get the help and encouragement of those you're motivating. It's a wonderful circle.

Where Do You Start?

How people make changes has been studied closely. It may help you to know the stages of change, so you can see where you are. If you're not even thinking about making a change, it just isn't going to happen. According to Debbie Dudley, RN, CDE, the stages of change progress as follows:

1. Not even thinking about making the change.
2. Thinking about making the change.
3. Getting ready to make the change.
4. Making the change.
5. Still making the change.
6. Not making the change anymore—the change has been made.

You won't change until something gets your attention and makes you want to change. Maybe your marriage is a little rocky right now, or your cousin tells you how much weight you've gained, or your high school reunion is coming, or your child is getting married and you want to look good in the pictures. All of these things can be wake-up calls. Once you become aware of your true condition, you can get motivated to change it for the better.

Knowledge is power. You need to know what actions will work for you. Step back for a second and *honestly* answer the following questions:

1. Do you try to convince yourself that your health issues aren't serious?
2. Do you feel like a victim?
3. Are you in denial about what you need to do for yourself?
4. Are you depressed or angry?
5. Are you absorbed in your own problems and never think of others?

If you answered yes to some of these questions (and most of us, if we are being honest with ourselves, will), then you have recognized some of the signs that you are getting in your own way. You are defeating all the good that you could be doing for yourself.

Write Around the Problem to Get to the Solution

Do you keep a journal? Writing about yourself works for almost everyone. You can write about your fears, your questions, what works, and what doesn't. Write about a bad day so you can learn from it. Write what happened and what you feel about it. Write about your viewpoint, and then try to take the other person's viewpoint, too. Write about your attitudes and whether they helped you in this situation. Write about your health choices and how they are making you feel, physically, mentally, and spiritually.

If you're having trouble, write about what you think is stopping you from reaching your goal. If you are in denial, or angry, or hopeless about your physical condition, your emotions are getting in your way. Feelings affect what you do or don't do.

Your journal might help you see what is preventing you from reaching your goal. You might brainstorm solutions

Barriers to Behavior Change	
Behavior	**Example**
Denial	"Why should I listen? This doesn't apply to me."
Anger	"I didn't have a choice. I don't want this disease. It's not fair!"
Comfort	"I like doing things the same old way."
Hopeless	"I can't control it. All my relatives died of this."
Tradition	"Nobody in my family ever did these things."
Fear	"What if I can't do this? What if I hurt myself? What if other people leave me because I'm too much trouble?"
Failure	"It doesn't matter what I do, I always fail."

with your family, friends, and health care providers. We all need some help sometime. If you're ready to move, get help.

Write about anyone who inspires you. Who inspires you to try something new?

Hang around with that person more. Read about people who have succeeded at what you want to do.

"What about Us?"

Be aware that when you start changing your behavior at home, the other members of the family are going to be uncomfortable. Now they have to change, too. They may be upset with you, even though you are doing healthy things for yourself and everybody else in the family. They may even try to subconsciously sabotage your new lifestyle through ridicule or criticism. It's not that they don't love you or don't want you to succeed. It's just that they have not resolved themselves as you have, and they may not be ready for

Some Healthy Thoughts to Try on for Size

- Eat to heal your body, not to entertain your mouth. A better way to entertain your mouth is to sing a song or pay someone a compliment. Very often, the act of snacking represents unconscious eating. We act like those calories don't count. They do!
- Laughter lowers your blood pressure and your blood sugar. It's exercise for the heart and soul!
- To be well it is important to think happy thoughts. Instead of flipping on evening news when you get home, play some music every once in awhile.

change. Tell them why you are changing and how proud you are to be doing it. Set a good example and let them follow in their own good time.

Addictions

Every human has the opportunity to become addicted to one thing or another. Some of us just don't; we have other challenges. Some of us are addicted to alcohol, tobacco, or drugs. Some people are addicted to sex. Some have become addicted to food; though, since eating food is legal and necessary for life, it falls into a special category. You can't quit food "cold turkey" like you can alcohol or tobacco. You have to eat. But you can *use* food for purposes other than sustenance, and that's when it's an addiction. People get addicted to food because the feeling they have while they're eating is the feeling of being loved.

Maybe that's why people get addicted to anything—it makes them feel loved. But if you look at it in the light of day, this is not love. "Things" can't love you. And do you really love something that damages or destroys you, as addictions do? Let me quote Dr. Andrew Weil on addictions. He says,

> Ironically, whatever satisfaction we gain from food, drugs, sex, money, or other "sources" of pleasure really comes from inside us. We project our power onto external substances and activities, allowing them to make us feel better temporarily. This is a strange sort of magic. We give our power away in order to achieve a transient sense of wholeness, then suffer because the objects of our craving seem to have power over us. (*Natural Health, Natural Medicine*, pp. 148–149)

There are real ways to feel loved. Help someone else. Give someone—preferably someone you live with—a sincere compliment every day. Get a pet and take good care of him. Find out what your strengths are and use them.

Make no mistake, eating too much is as damaging to your health as too much tobacco, alcohol, or drugs. If you have the challenge of an addiction, you also have the opportunity to find out why you're addicted and to do something about it. You can make a different choice and see what happens to you.

There are short-term therapies for behavior change or cognitive changes dealing with addiction. You might look into one of these to help you find the triggers and build new responses to them. Body therapies, such as massage and acupuncture, help with conquering addiction, when you are ready to change. Exercise, such as walking and yoga, certainly help your body feel calmer and deal with the stress of making such an important change.

Trading in Your Habits

We've talked a lot about making changes. Let's look at the other side of the coin: habits. In a lot of ways, dealing with a habit is a lot like dealing with an addiction. Instead of facing an issue, you turn to what's comfortable instead of what may be the best option. People fall into habits so they don't have to make choices every day. That's the lazy way to go through life, and those habits cost you spontaneity and fun and maybe some better choices.

When you make new choices, unusual choices, different choices, you give yourself a treat. You wake yourself up. Pay attention to the choices you make at each moment. Don't do something merely because it's the way you've always done it. Maybe there's a better way, or maybe just thinking about it helps you see that your way really is the best way after all.

What You Can Do

If you are only willing to make just one change in your life, let me make a suggestion: add a daily walk. Your goal should

---

Prayer Works

Some of you may already know that prayer works to help people heal. Some of you may just hope it does. But in the past few years, more and more medical institutions, such as Duke, Harvard, and the Mayo Clinic, are doing research to try and measure how effective prayer is. The National Institute of Health (NIH) and Johns Hopkins University are looking into it as well. From individuals praying in other countries to support group prayers for breast cancer survivors, there is mounting evidence that praying for people helps them get better. And in fact, when you are a member of a church or group that prays for others, you are likely to be healthier, too. Remember that people who go to church actually have been found to live longer.

be to walk for 30 minutes to an hour—even if you start by walking down the driveway to the mailbox. Stay after it, and that one change will make a big difference in your health, your mood, and your life.

If you are feeling adventurous and you are willing to make *two* changes, I have another suggestion: reduce sugar-containing sodas and drinks in favor of diet sodas and flavored waters.

If you are truly a brave soul and you're willing to make *three* changes, add four or five vegetables to your day.

With these three seemingly simple changes, you can revolutionize your life. If you don't believe me, just try and see for yourself. You've got nothing to lose and the rest of your life to gain.

Whatever You Do, Deal with Stress

Stress is an important part of life. Stress is good when it helps us build mental and physical muscle. Without stress, you wouldn't know how strong you are. Stress is bad when you can't figure out how to get away from it. Instead of strengthening yourself, you eat, drink, or smoke too much to try and turn it off. Have these helped so far? I can tell you right now that other than for a few fleeting moments, none of those methods ever will.

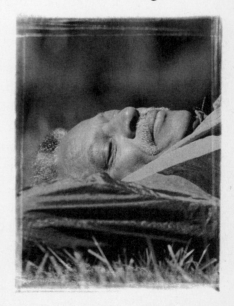

Healthy ways of relieving stress are exercise, yoga, meditation, prayer, and deep breathing. We can measure the effects of these methods on the body through blood pressure, muscle tension, and heart rate. These mindful methods trigger the

---

Quick Stress Reliever

One of the easiest methods of relieving stress is to simply breathe. Sit up straight in a quiet place. Take a slow deep breath to the count of four. Hold it for a count of four. Exhale slowly for a count of four. Recognize any thoughts that want to intervene and let them go. Return to your breath and your count. Don't think about what happened yesterday that upset you, and don't think about what is going to happen tomorrow. Just sit and breathe. Be mindful of where you are right now and what you are doing. This makes your mind and your body calmer.

When you're upset, or under attack, or can't think what to do, breathe.

---

relaxation response in your body and make it healthier. Research is just now scratching the surface of how much healthier these activities make us, but we have studies that show its beneficial effect on heart disease, blood pressure, chronic pain, menopause symptoms, and insomnia, among others.

Regular exercise relieves stress by working your muscles (especially your heart) so they can relax. It also releases endorphins, feel-good hormones in the brain, that relax you and make you feel good. Yoga is a combination of tensing and relaxing muscles and breathing consciously. This is why it is singled out as being one of the most effective ways to relieve stress.

Being mindful of the present moment, no matter what you are doing, is actually calming. Even if you are in pain or uncomfortable, it is just this one moment you are focused on. The next one will be different in some way, and you will see that when it arrives. This act of concentration, called mindfulness meditation, is being studied now because it appears to change the mental outlook of the people who practice it. Mindful meditation, such as that taught by Jon Kabat-Zinn and others, has been shown to relieve stress and to encourage this shift in attitude. Not a bad return for a few moments of your time each day.

More Stress Relievers
Exercise
Yoga
Mindfulness meditation
Prayer
Good night's sleep

Resources

Online

The following websites offer meditation tapes that can help to calm you and relieve stress:

Mind/Body Medical Institute
www.mbmi.org

The Center for Mindfulness
www.umassmed.edu/cfm

Jon Kabat-Zinn
www.mindfulnesstapes.com

Associations

Center for Mental Health Services
Knowledge Exchange Network
P.O. Box 42557
Washington, D.C. 20015
800-789-2647
www.mentalhealth.org

Alcoholics Anonymous (AA)
Grand Central Station
Box 459
New York, NY 10163
212-870-3400
www.aa.org

Substance Abuse and Mental Health
Services Administration
Room 12-105 Parklawn Building
5600 Fishers Lane
Rockville, MD 20857
301-443-8956
www.samhsa.gov

**National Clearinghouse for Alcohol
and Drug Information**
P.O. Box 2345
Rockville, MD 20847-2345
800-729-6686
800-4889 TTY
www.health.org

HHS Center for Faith-Based and Community Initiatives
200 Independence Avenue, SW
Washington, D.C. 20201
877-696-6775
www.hhs.gov/faith

Books

Acts of Faith, by Iyanla Vanzant, Simon and Schuster, 1993. This is a daily meditation book for people of color.

Saving Our Last Nerve: The Black Woman's Path to Mental Health, by Marilyn Martin, MD, MPH. Hilton Publishing, 2002.

Diabetes Burnout, by William Polonsky, PhD. American Diabetes Association, 1998.

Also available on audio tape. This book has light-hearted but useful sections on why people don't exercise or take care of their diabetes and what to do about them. Great introduction to behavior change for better health.

Audio Book:

Three Levels of Power and How to Use Them, Carolyn Myss, PhD, Sounds True, 1997. Can be ordered from *www.soundstrue.com*.

5

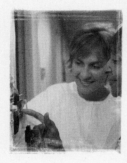

OVERWEIGHT AND OBESITY

We're all trying to get to a healthy weight. The problem is that not everyone knows what a healthy weight is. A healthy weight doesn't mean a pretty weight. It doesn't mean you have to be stick thin. A healthy weight is just what the name implies—the weight at which you have normal blood pressure, normal blood sugar, normal cholesterol, and your ankles and knees aren't hurting. See what I mean about a healthy weight? A healthy weight doesn't mean looking like a lollipop with a stick body and big round head. A healthy weight prevents complications, and means you're healthier all over.

This raises a question, though: Is your weight a problem for you? If you don't think it is, then you're not going to make any changes. But think about it a bit. Are you tired of not finding clothes to fit you, or of having to buy new ones because the old ones are too small? Are you tired of being out of

Obesity Leads To:	
• High blood pressure	• Arthritis
• High cholesterol	• Gallstones
• Heart disease	• Asthma
• Stroke	• Depression
• Insulin resistance	• Sleep apnea and snoring
• Diabetes	

breath from doing even the smallest physical activity or of not having any energy to do anything? Are you having problems fitting into your car or a seat at the movies? If so, let's talk about what you can do to lose some weight. You can do it, but first, you have to decide that you really want to. Being ready to change counts most in your success.

Being overweight can do a powerful awful thing to your body. It works quite a number on the joints in your back and legs and feet. Do yours hurt? And that's nothing compared to what's being done on the inside.

A Growing Problem

The number one health threat in the U.S. is obesity and lack of fitness. It now kills as many as smoking. Half of all the adults in the U.S. are overweight or obese. And the kids are catching up fast. Obesity has doubled in the U.S. in the past 25 years. It has tripled in adolescents.

Obesity is causing a rise in new cases of diabetes, too. The number of Americans with diabetes has risen 50% in 10 years, with a million new cases diagnosed each year. Obesity is why the children are developing type 2 diabetes, which up until the last ten years was a disease of middle-aged or elderly people. Nearly 9 million kids are seriously overweight. They are developing adult diseases that are directly caused by what they eat and the exercise they are not doing. This simply can't go on like this.

"Healthy" Body Image?

It's funny what people will study, but a recent poll showed that 67% of African Americans like the way they look and are comfortable with their bodies. This is twice as high as the next nearest group. That speaks well for our self-image. It may not speak well for our waist size, however. We may be so okay with ourselves that a lot of us don't feel compelled to lose the weight we need to lose. While I'd never want to convince anyone to not be happy with themselves, I think it's time we recognized what is good for our bodies. Loving yourself is wonderful, but are you really loving yourself if your lifestyle is bad for you? You don't want to hurt the ones you love, especially if that person is yourself. Be good to yourself. You only have one body. Make the most of it.

Open your hand and take hold of your belly or your thigh. Is it ample and soft? Some people call this fat. It's really stored energy. It is food you have eaten that you didn't use, and it will stay there until you burn it in exercise. That extra energy is not good, even when it's in pretty places.

Where Are You Now?

Nobody sets out with a goal to get fat and be unhealthy. You just go along from day to day and for one reason or another—the kids make fun of you on the playground, or your cousin can't help being honest about how big you are—you get a wake-up call. If you don't set any goals for yourself, this is where you wind up: Overweight, diagnosed with diabetes, in grave danger of heart attack and stroke.

You can just ignore it and wait for the worst to happen. Or you can think about your choices and see which ones you might like to try.

One Woman's Story

"I didn't realize I was putting on so much weight. Just one day the waistband of my skirt was too tight, so I bought a larger size. And then a larger size. I'll admit it, I usually wear a 10, but I was up to an 18. Still, I didn't think too much of it until I saw my cousin at an annual family birthday party. She took one look at me and said, "Oh, girl, you've gained another person!" When I looked hurt, she tried to make it better, but I couldn't ignore the fact that I had gained a lot of weight, and it showed to everyone but me.

My feelings were hurt, and I kept replaying the look on her face and what she said. Finally, I decided to do something instead of sitting there and whining about it.

I signed up for a "boot camp" at a local gym. Boot camp is all about teamwork, and I had my team members to help me keep going. It was four days a week, an hour a day, which isn't much, but I lost seven pounds in that month. I felt so good about myself. I escaped the "poor me" and was feeling better and looking better. I've kept up the walking and eating smaller-sized meals, and it's working. Now I wish I'd saved some of those beautiful outfits I used to fit into. I'm ready for them now."

What Is a Reasonable Weight for You?

Before you set any goals, determining how much you should weigh is a priority. Overweight and obesity are measured by the numbers on the BMI scale, which are derived from a comparison of height and weight. The numbers on the scale generally range from 19 to 40, with 19 being the lightest and 40 being the heaviest. A healthy weight is a BMI of somewhere between 21 and 24. Overweight is a BMI of 25 to 29.9. Obesity is a BMI of 30 or higher.

To figure out your BMI, look at Figure 5-1. BMI Chart on page 108. Find your height in inches on the left hand column and scan across to the right until you find your weight. This weight will be listed under a number at the very top of the column. This is your BMI. For example, a man who is five-foot-nine (69 inches) and weighs 189 pounds has a BMI of 28. This is overweight, but not quite obese.

Overweight means you weigh too much for your height, but this is not an exact gauge of how much extra fat you have. That extra weight could be muscle, bone, and water, as well as fat. Professional football players, for example, weigh more than non-athletes of the same height because they have more muscle mass. Chances are, though, you're not a professional football player and any extra weight you're carrying around is in the form of fat, not well-developed muscle.

The BMI chart gives you an idea of reasonable body weights for your specific height. You and your doctor need to decide what is reasonable for you. We know that at the far ends of this scale—for very short or very tall people—the chart is not accurate, but it helps give you an idea of where you are and where you may want to go.

Waist High

Of course, how much you actually weigh is not the only thing to focus on. You should also be aware of where the obesity is. Obesity around your waist is more dangerous than obesity on your hips and thighs. This is actually as good a measure of your health risks as the BMI. All doctors should carry a tape-measure; I do. If your navel enters my office before your nose does, then you have a problem. Get the picture?

Measure your waist. If it is greater than 40 inches for men and 35 inches for women, you have central obesity. It's in the center of you, where all your vital organs are. Men patients often tell me that their belt size is 34, so they can't have this

Body Mass Index (BMI) Values

BMI

	Good Weights								Increasing Risk													
Height	**19**	**20**	**21**	**22**	**23**	**24**	**25**	**26**	**27**	**28**	**29**	**30**	**31**	**32**	**33**	**34**	**35**	**36**	**37**	**38**	**39**	**40**
										Weight (in pounds)												
4'10"	91	96	100	105	110	115	119	124	129	134	138	143	148	153	158	162	167	172	177	181	186	191
4'11"	94	99	104	109	114	119	124	128	133	138	143	148	153	158	163	168	173	178	183	188	193	198
5'	97	102	107	112	118	123	128	133	138	143	148	153	158	163	168	174	179	184	189	194	199	204
5'1"	100	106	111	116	122	127	132	137	143	148	153	158	164	169	174	180	185	190	195	201	206	211
5'2"	104	109	115	120	126	131	136	142	147	153	158	164	169	175	180	186	191	196	202	207	213	218
5'3"	107	113	118	124	130	135	141	146	152	158	163	169	175	180	186	191	197	203	208	214	220	225
5'4"	110	116	122	128	134	140	145	151	157	163	169	174	180	186	192	197	204	209	215	221	227	232
5'5"	114	120	126	132	138	144	150	156	162	168	174	180	186	192	198	204	210	216	222	228	234	240
5'6"	118	124	130	136	142	148	155	161	167	173	179	186	192	198	204	210	216	223	229	235	241	247
5'7"	121	127	134	140	146	153	159	166	172	178	185	191	198	204	211	217	223	230	236	242	249	255
5'8"	125	131	138	144	151	158	164	171	177	184	190	197	203	210	216	223	230	236	243	249	256	262
5'9"	128	135	142	149	155	162	169	176	182	189	196	203	209	216	223	230	236	243	250	257	263	270
5'10"	132	139	146	153	160	167	174	181	188	195	202	209	216	222	229	236	243	250	257	264	271	278
5'11"	136	143	150	157	165	172	179	186	193	200	208	215	222	229	236	243	250	257	265	272	279	286
6'	140	147	154	162	169	177	184	191	199	206	213	221	228	235	242	250	258	265	272	279	287	294
6'1"	144	151	159	166	174	182	189	197	204	212	219	227	235	242	250	257	265	272	280	288	295	302
6'2"	148	155	163	171	179	186	194	202	210	218	225	233	241	249	256	264	272	280	287	295	303	311
6'3"	152	160	168	176	184	192	200	208	216	224	232	240	248	256	264	272	279	287	295	303	311	319
6'4"	156	164	172	180	189	197	205	213	221	230	238	246	254	263	271	279	287	295	304	312	320	328

BMI ≥27 are highlighted because health risk escalates rapidly above this level.

problem. Yes, their belt size hasn't changed since high school, but their belly sure has. The belt just fits down underneath it now. Be honest and measure across your waist where the belly button is. Or at least where it is supposed to be.

When you're thick through the middle, your body can't use insulin properly, and your organs get very crowded. This condition is the single largest cause of heart attacks, heart disease, and death. It is preventable and treatable.

Cholesterol

There are two kinds of cholesterol, HDL (good) and LDL (bad). As you can imagine, if you're overweight or obese you've probably got a lot of LDL running around in your system, and not a lot of HDL.

If you can get your HDL (good) cholesterol above 60, you could cut your chances of having a heart attack six-fold. How do you increase HDL levels? Exercise, quitting alcohol, quitting smoking, and losing weight. But the greatest of these is exercise. The effect of exercise on your HDL is simple. If you exercise some, you get some improvement in HDL. If you exercise like an Olympic athlete, you get the highest HDL levels of all. Triathletes have the next highest HDL levels and so on, down to the low HDL of that person sitting on the couch.

Hey, you on the couch, you can't change your genes, but you can change your HDL levels. And save yourself from the experience of a heart attack. You're never too old to turn off the TV and go outside and play.

If your LDL cholesterol is still too high, you can take a statin to bring it down. These are very effective drugs. If you don't like taking drugs, you can take it for awhile, until you can change some of your eating and exercise habits so you can lose some weight. Your blood pressure and cholesterol levels will come down naturally, and you may not need the drug any longer. A side effect of taking a statin can be muscle pain. If you are taking the drug and begin to be more active at the same time, you may think you're exercising too much and stop, when in fact, it is a side effect of the drug. Talk with your doctor about what to do and ask what medication might be best for you.

Insulin Resistance

Remember I said that people who are obese around the middle have a problem using the insulin that their body makes. The body resists the action of the insulin, so the pancreas has to make more and more insulin to try to get the glucose out of the bloodstream. People with insulin resistance have higher than normal blood sugar levels, but not as high as in diabetes. Doesn't matter if you're all the way to diabetes, yet. Insulin resistance and high blood sugar damage your heart and blood vessels just like diabetes does. The conditions that raise your chances of having insulin resistance are obesity, not exercising, going through puberty, and having polycystic ovary disease. Being African American or Latino increases your chance of having it, too.

You can see that your overweight children, particularly your daughters, have a chance of developing insulin resistance, Metabolic Syndrome, and worse. Help them. Puberty is a time of insulin resistance. I know that the teenage years are a time of resisting everything, but even kids who are not overweight have lower insulin sensitivity during puberty. They all need to eat better and to get some exercise.

Taking Control

If you are overweight or obese, take heart, because the news isn't all bad. There is one very positive aspect to being too heavy—it is curable. You can lose weight and you can keep it off. By doing so, you're treating one condition and preventing a bunch of much meaner ones.

Be Active

Eating is less of a problem if you exercise. Like I've said before, I'm not going to fuss at you so much about your eating if you exercise. If you love to eat and you love good food, you don't have to give it all up (though you may want to love it in less amounts from now on). Just get out there and burn it off. To put it another way, if you choose only one thing to change, choose exercise. For more ideas on what you can do to start burning off that extra fuel, go back and look at Chapter 3. Being Active Is Being Alive.

Be Patient

If you are overweight, it took you years to get there. Please don't try to take it all off in one month. Whatever you do, don't starve yourself. Here's the thing about starvation diets: if you don't eat, your metabolism slows down. This is a safety mechanism to save your life during a famine. Your body doesn't know that you're starving on purpose. It can't believe you would actually do that. Most often, the weight you lose during a starvation diet is water weight, instead of actual fat. You may weigh less, but you're not thinner and you haven't lost any weight.

Eat. You can still lose weight. You just need smaller serving sizes. Have you ever measured your servings? You might be amazed to find that what you call one serving of rice is actually enough for five people. Check Chapter 2. Real Food, for suggestions on how much is a good serving.

Stop Weighing Yourself Every Day

This sounds crazy, doesn't it? How are you going to know if you've lost any weight if you don't weigh yourself? Believe me, you'll know. The notches in your belt and the reflection in the mirror will start to tell you. Being able to breathe when you get to the top of the staircase will let you know.

The problem with weighing yourself on a scale everyday is that your weight fluctuates all the time, sometimes by as much as a few pounds a day. Weighing yourself on a day to day basis isn't a good gauge for how much real weight you're actually losing. This is why those two-week crash diets seem to work so well. They make you lose weight—mostly water weight—but not any fat. The scale may say you've lost 10 pounds, but you haven't lost it where it matters. As soon as you quit the diet (and you *will* quit the diet. You can't starve yourself forever), all that weight comes back almost immediately.

So instead of weighing yourself every morning and night, weigh yourself once every two weeks, or once a month. Not only does this give you a better gauge of how much weight you are really losing, it also puts your goals into the proper perspective. Getting control of overweight and obesity is not a fourteen-day job. You're in it for the long haul. Thinking on a month to month timeline, instead of day to day, will make this easier.

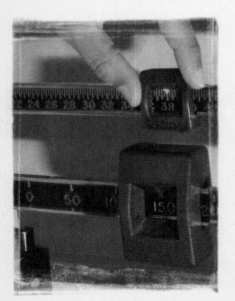

Obesity Drugs

There is no drug or herb or vitamin that magically causes weight loss. If you don't use good food choices, smaller servings, and a daily walk, it just isn't going to happen. That's the secret. However, if you have a BMI of 30 or greater, and you have started a program of eating better and exercise, weight-loss drugs might help support your efforts. The drugs most often prescribed are Xenical, Meridia, and Ionamin or Adipex-P. Xenical has shown up in a research study as helping to prevent heart attacks in people who take it to help lose weight. If you are obese and have diabetes, your chance of a heart attack is high, so you and your doctor may want to discuss this drug for you.

If you don't lose weight in the first two or three months, then the drugs don't work for you. These drugs are very powerful and have side effects that you may not want to have. Also, most insurance companies won't pay for weight-loss drugs. Don't despair. The most powerful tools are in your hands already. Your efforts with food and exercise will pay off. Your dedication will be the deciding factor—not a pill.

Other drugs suppress appetite with amphetamines. People can get addicted to these drugs, so they are not recommended. Some folks also try diuretics and laxatives to lose weight. The weight you lose, however, is once again water weight, which you'll gain back when you come to your senses and have a glass of water.

Surgery for Obesity—A Last Resort

With a well-known TV weatherman and a rock royalty pop singer having surgery to lose weight, a lot of folks may be thinking about having that surgery to make their stomachs smaller. Think about surgery as the last resort. After the surgery, you do have to make changes to your lifestyle or the weight can come back—even if your stomach is much smaller. This procedure is appropriate for people with a BMI greater than 40, or a BMI of 35 if they also have a condition like diabetes that will improve from the surgery.

The small stomach pouch that is created in the surgery can only hold a cup of food. That's the secret. You just eat less. I suggest you save the thousands of dollars and just eat less on your own without the surgery and see how much weight you can lose that way.

Most patients lose about 100 pounds in the year after surgery. This significant weight loss lowers blood pressure, ends snoring and sleep apnea, improves heart health, and relieves arthritis pain. Blood sugar levels come down. There are, however, a lot of Ifs to consider before scheduling the surgery. If you have tried very-low-calorie diets and exercise and have not been able to get your BMI down from 40, and if your doctor agrees that the surgery would help lower your health risks, and if your insurance company is willing to cover the procedure, then you might check with the American Society for Bariatric Surgery (*www.asbs.org*) to find a qualified surgeon.

My concern is about the side effects of the surgery, such as gallstones and depression, and the fact that your digestive system is forever going to be abnormal. Don't take this idea lightly. You'll be unable to absorb nutrients from food through normal digestion and will have to take vitamin and mineral supplements for the rest of your life. Please find out everything about the surgery and its side effects before you start weighing the pros and cons of having it done to you. Also be sure to find a surgeon who is experienced in doing this type of surgery and a practice that will support you through the surgery and for the years after.

One last point; the actor Stephen Furst (Flounder on *Animal House*) designed his own low-fat diet and lost 75 pounds in the first year of eating the new way. This is as much weight lost as the surgery provides! His sister had gastric bypass surgery and lost 150 pounds, only to put the weight back on again. She did this by drinking lots of milk-shakes and sugary drinks that packed a lot of calories. Stephen accomplished the same weight loss—his final total weight lost was 150 pounds—without surgery. Think about it. Wouldn't you like to try your own plan first?

What Helps You Succeed

The National Weight Control Registry (NWCR) is a large study in the U.S. that follows people who have successfully lost weight. Most of the people on the registry have lost about 60 pounds and have kept it off for more than five years. Nearly three quarters of them were overweight in childhood or the teen years. Almost all had tried to lose weight before and gained it back again. That seems to be the biggest problem; keeping the weight from coming back.

What are the roads to success with weight loss? Here's some advice from the people in the registry:

- Get professional help from Weight Watchers or a dietitian. You need to know what healthy food choices are.

- Change both your eating and your activity levels.

- Eat smaller amounts, develop your own menus, or follow an Exchange meal plan.

- Eat regular meals and snacks. Don't skip breakfast.

- Eat out only occasionally. Learn which foods are your best choices when you do eat out.

- Be active every day, with a goal of one hour of brisk walking or biking or other activity.

- Weigh once a week or once a month, but not more often.

- Get less calories from saturated fat—remember to eat good fats!

Most said that they succeeded because they had a strong reason for making the commitment to get healthier. The ones who lost weight on their own, without an organized program like Weight Watchers, found it was easier to keep the weight off than the people in structured programs or on special foods. When you make a plan for yourself, it fits you best. The longer they followed a healthy lifestyle, the easier it was to maintain the weight loss. Does this sound like common sense to you?

When you accept the challenge of losing weight, you can focus on making a plan that fits your life and the way you do things. You know that you have to change both what and how often you eat, but you can also have dessert every now and then. You know that you have to be more active every day. Variety in foods and in exercise keeps you entertained and motivated. Perhaps, most important is learning to deal with your problems instead of eating to forget or escape them.

What about All These Diets?

So many people get tempted by the idea of a diet that lets you eat everything and still lose weight. In your heart, you know that doesn't make good sense. You don't need a fancy-pants diet, but if you're curious about them, here's what the experts say. The United States Department of Agriculture (USDA) and the Physicians Committee for Responsible Medicine (PCRM) rated the most popular diets on how healthy they are as a way to eat for the rest of your life. PCRM liked diets with:

- 25 grams of fiber a day (from fruits, vegetables, and whole grains)

- 5 or more servings of fruit and vegetables a day

- Less than 300 milligrams of cholesterol a day

- Fewer than 30% of calories from fat

- Fewer than 10% of calories from saturated fats.

They gave the popular diets a rating from 0 to 5 stars. Then they rated diets as either acceptable or unacceptable. The results of both are shown in Table 5-1. What about All These Diet Books?

What the USDA Says

The USDA report in the March 2001 issue of *Obesity Research* used the same diet guidelines as the PCRM—more fiber, less saturated fat, and 5-a-day fruit and vegetables. Based on strong scientific evidence, they recommend a moderate-fat, balanced diet. This is the type of diet you find in programs such as Weight Watchers. This is the meal plan you can build using the Food Guide Pyramid, the cholesterol-lowering Step I and Step II Diets, and the blood pressure-lowering DASH diet. See Chapter 2 for more help with what to eat.

Metabolic Syndrome or Syndrome X

Sounds like science fiction, doesn't it? Syndrome X, or the Metabolic Syndrome, sounds bad. It is. It means that your digestive and metabolic system, which takes in food and turns out energy to keep your body working right, is out of order. Who has it? You do if you are overweight and you also have high blood pressure and high cholesterol or high blood sugar. Three strikes and you're out. While the Metabolic Syndrome is not "contagious" in the strictest sense of the word, you and your children can "catch" it by gaining weight.

Why do you care if you have Metabolic Syndrome? Medical research shows that you are three times more likely to have heart disease and to die early. Metabolic syndrome is a killer, but like obesity, it responds very well to treatment. You can escape it. You can prevent your children from developing it. Drop the sugary drinks. Start walking.

Table 5-1. What about All These Diet Books?

Star ratings are from the Physicians Committee for Responsible Medicine (PCRM) May 2000 report. Acceptable and unacceptable ratings are from a January 2001 PCRM press release.

Title	Author	Ratings
Dr. Atkins New Diet Revolution	R. Atkins	0 stars, Unacceptable
Protein Power	M. Eades and M.D. Eades	Unacceptable
The Carbohydrate Addict's Lifespan Program	R. Heller and R. Heller	0 stars
The Carbohydrate Addict's Diet	R. Heller and R. Heller	Unacceptable
Dieting for Dummies	J. Kirby	3 stars
Eat More, Weigh Less	D. Ornish	5 stars, Acceptable
Body for Life	B. Phillips	2 stars
Volumetrics	B. Rolls and R.A. Barnett	Acceptable
The Soy Zone	B. Sears	3 stars
The Zone	B. Sears	Acceptable
Dr. Shapiro's Picture Perfect Weight Loss	H.M. Shapiro	4 stars
Sugar Busters!	H.L. Steward, S.S. Andrews, M.C. Bethea, and L.A. Balart	2 stars, Unacceptable
Dieting with the Duchess	Sarah, Duchess of York, and Weight Watchers	Acceptable
Weight Watchers: New Complete Cookbook	Weight Watchers	3 stars
Eating Well for Optimum Health	A. Weil	4 stars

The Levels You Want to Reach	
Waist measurement (around the belly-button, remember?)	Less than 40 inches for men Less than 35 for women
Triglycerides	Less than 150
HDL Cholesterol	Greater than 50 for women Greater than 40 for men
Blood Pressure	120/80 or lower
Blood Glucose	Fasting glucose less than 110

Your chances of getting Syndrome X are increased by your age and the genes that you inherit. Males over 50 and females over 60 have a greater chance of developing this condition. Right now in the United States, about half of all people in their 50s have Metabolic Syndrome. You can't change your age or your genes. But you can change your exercise and eating habits, which will change your cholesterol, blood pressure, and blood sugar levels.

After taking these lifestyle steps, if you still have high blood pressure or high cholesterol or high blood sugar, there are drugs to lower these levels. You do have the tools to escape Syndrome X if you are willing to use them. You have the power to make amazing changes in your health.

To Treat Metabolic Syndrome

The way to treat the Metabolic Syndrome is the same as the way to treat overweight and obesity. Eat fewer calories and exercise daily to burn up the calories you do eat. It's really not any more complicated than that. Burn more than you eat, lose weight, and your body will start taking care of itself.

The Children Follow

Children have a knack for picking up their parents' habits, both good and bad. When you are overweight, your children are more likely to be overweight. There are a lot of social forces involved in weight gain, but you are still the single biggest influence in your child's life. Obesity usually runs in the family. You may tell your child that he needs to lose a few pounds, but unless he sees you trying to do the same thing he's probably not going to change his ways.

Overweight Children Break My Heart

I can show you pictures and case study after case study of children who have lost their childhood because they are so overweight. The 5-year-old girl who weighs 150 pounds and can't even wear children's clothes. The 16-year-old boy who weighs 530 pounds. Trying out for the track or soccer team is not an option. Getting a good night's sleep is not an option.

These children have the same problems with obesity that adults do. They snore, which is a sign they have sleep apnea. They can't breathe while they sleep, so they are not getting the oxygen they need to be rested when they wake up. They are sleepy all day and not able to pay attention at school. They've already got self-image problems without feeling bad about being poor students, too. A child with sleep apnea may fall asleep in the car on a short ride. She may have morning headaches or wet the bed. He may behave badly or be too cranky to cooperate with others. Losing weight returns the joy of sleeping to your child.

I know of one obese teenager who had to sleep sitting up with his head against the wall. That wasn't what worried his parents, though. They brought him to see the doctor because there was dark brown, velvety skin on the back of his neck. This velvety skin is called acanthosis nigricans and is a signal that the obese child has insulin resistance.

You can see the dark patches and the obesity. What you can't see that is just as real is the damage being done to your child's heart, liver, lungs, and gallbladder. An obese child has a grown-up chance of heart disease, stroke, arthritis, diabetes, liver damage, depression, asthma, and cancer.

What Can You Do?

Look at what your children are eating. Do their daily meals come from the four "kid" food groups (see the box "The Four 'Kid' Food Groups")?

Research shows that kids who drink sugary beverages, such as soda, fruit punch, bottled tea, or drinks made from fruit-flavored powders, take in too many calories. Kids pass up milk and water if sweet drinks are offered or available. The Center for Science in the Public Interest calls soft drinks "liquid candy" because they are the biggest source of refined sugar in the American diet. In fact, 12- to 19-year-old boys get almost half of their 34 teaspoons of sugar a day from soft drinks.

Our genes never thought we were going to drink our calories. There are five things you can do to help your children right now.

1. Don't bring home the sodas, the cereals, or the candy with so much sugar in them.

The Four "Kid" Food Groups

- Soft drinks (sodas, sports drinks, drink mixes)
- Fast foods (McDonalds, Burger King, Wendy's, Taco Bell, KFC)
- Sugared cereals (Fruit Loops, Cocoa Puffs)
- Candy (Nerds, Snickers, Hersheys, M&Ms)

—Stephen W. Ponder, MD, CDE

2. If you do bring soda home, buy diet, and watch out for Gatorade and fruit juice, too.

3. Help your children drink 6 to 8 glasses of water a day.

4. Bring home fresh fruit and vegetables and whole grain cereals and crackers.

5. Buy them all pedometers and help them get 10,000 steps a day.

Soups and salads are the secret to success. You can put all kinds of chopped-up vegetables in soups and salads. Salad is very interesting with fruit, olives, a sprinkle of nuts, and a little grated cheese, too. Soups and salads are a great way into the world of vegetables. But watch the salad dressing—it's probably loaded with fat and calories. Olive oil or canola oil should be the base and there should always be moderation with salad dressing.

Fruit Kids Like	Veggies Kids Like
• Apple slices with peanut butter • Bananas (dip in chocolate sauce and freeze) • Kiwi • Watermelon • Strawberries • Grapes • Oranges • Canned peaches in light syrup, pineapple, and mixed fruit	• Corn • Broccoli with cheese sauce • Cucumbers • Carrots • Potatoes • Salad

How Does It Happen?

Most pediatricians do not discuss a child's weight with the parents. You and I need to discuss how children get obese and what you can do to protect your children from it. Understanding how a problem happens is the first step to correcting it. Most overweight children:

- Start gaining weight between 3 and 5 years of age

- Often eat fast food (and usually eat food fast!)

- Drink most of their extra calories

- May skip one or more meals a day and then graze all evening

- Watch 4 or more hours of TV a day

- Are tall for their ages

Adapted from a chart by Stephen W. Ponder, MD, CDE.

When obese children are toddlers, they usually have a bottle of milk or juice or soda that they carry everywhere. That's too many calories every day. When they switch to solid foods, they eat the food that is offered to them, just like they did with the bottle. Ask yourself these questions:

- Are you giving your child too much food?

- Are you allowing your child to drink too many sodas?

- Do you allow your child to eat from the time he gets home from school to the time he goes to bed?

- Do you allow your child to eat fast food every day?

- Do you use food as a reward for your child's good behavior?

- Are you using food to comfort your child when things go wrong?

- Do you set limits on TV and computer time?

- Do you encourage your child to be active and go participate in the activities?

How to Help and Support Your Child

Your overweight child does not need to be criticized, especially in front of others. Remember that he lives in a highly scrutinized world. More than likely, he wants this to be a private matter, so other people don't make fun of him or his efforts. He doesn't need more scrutiny, he needs you to help him set and reach some realistic goals. Together you can work on making the changes in eating and exercise that we discuss in this book. More often than not, if he sees you making the same efforts, he'll be much more open to changing his eating and exercise patterns. You need to be a role model. You should eat the same healthy foods and take a daily walk or swim or ride bikes with him. Be patient for him as you are for yourself. Everyone slips once in awhile. In fact, it may help to have a blow-out meal once in awhile. Be positive and believe he can do it. He can. And so can you.

A Few More Things to Consider

If you are an emotional eater, you might do better with a support group like TOPS (Take Off Pounds Sensibly) or Weight Watchers. Or start a weight loss club of your own. Avoid friends who encourage you to eat, or who drive you to overeating.

While you are working at losing weight, talk nicely about yourself—and to yourself. Encourage yourself. Don't beat yourself up. If you fall off the wagon, that's okay. Just start with healthier choices at the next meal.

Make soup. Make salad. Then you have days of healthy meals ready when you want them.

Only change one habit at a time. Add one vegetable at a time. Give yourself time. It took years to put the weight on, it may well take years to get all of it off. Losing 50 pounds a year is just fine. What am I saying? Fine? It's *wonderful*.

Visualize yourself the size you want to be. Get into all the details. What sports will you do? What new clothes will you buy? What will you like most about being thinner?

Resources

Associations

Weight Watchers International
800-972-7546
www.weightwatchers.com

Taking Off Pounds Sensibly (TOPS)
www.tops.org

Weight-control Information Network
1 WIN Way
Bethesda, MD 20892-3665
877-946-4627
www.niddk.nih.gov/health/nutrit/nutrit.htm

Books

Slim Down Sister, by Fabiola Demps Gaines, RD, LD, and Roniece Weaver, RD, LD, and Angela Ebron. Plume, 2001.

Month of Meals: Soul Food Selections, by Fabiola Demps Gaines, RD, LD, and Roniece Weaver, RD, LD. American Diabetes Association, 2003.

Confessions of a Couch Potato: Or If I'm So Skinny, Why Do I Still Feel Like Flounder? by Stephen Furst. American Diabetes Association, 2002.

Help! My Underwear is Shrinking, by JoAnn Hattner, Ann Coulston, Mike Goodkind. American Diabetes Association, 2003.

6

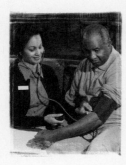

HIGH BLOOD PRESSURE

High blood pressure, also known as hypertension, affects about 50 million people in America—that's one in four adults. But this is no longer just an adult condition. These numbers are spilling over into younger and younger populations. In the growing number of obese children, high blood pressure has been showing up in kids as young as 7 years old. It is very common among African Americans, and we tend to develop it when we are younger. While high blood pressure itself is not debilitating, it is a sign that something much more serious is around the corner. It is a danger signal.

What Is Hypertension?

In general, blood pressure measures the force of the blood against the walls of the blood vessels. It is recorded as two numbers. The top number, called the systolic pressure, is measured when your heart beats. The bottom number, called the diastolic pressure, is measured when your heart is at rest in-between beats. Both numbers are important. The guideline for normal blood pressure is 120/80. Blood pressure that measures up to 139/89 is called prehypertension, which means that unless you do something soon, you will almost definitely develop high blood pressure. Blood pressures of 140/90 or higher show that you have hypertension. You need to bring it down.

Blood pressure naturally rises and falls over the day and night, but if it stays high all the time, it makes your heart work too hard. It exerts too much pressure on blood vessels all over your body, pushing them to their limits like water building in a clogged fire hose. And just like the fire hose, it has explosive power. This is why high blood pressure can cause heart attacks and strokes. Your kidneys are in danger, too (see Chapter 9).

If your parents or brothers and sisters have high blood pressure, you are more likely to have it. If you have diabetes, you are more likely to have it. If you are under a great deal of stress at work or home, and you don't know healthy ways to relieve the stress, you are more likely to have it, too.

But I Feel Fine

You may feel fine and have no symptoms and still have high blood pressure. It is often discovered on a routine office visit to the doctor. However, a single high blood pressure reading does not necessarily mean you have hypertension. Like I said, blood pressure naturally rises and falls due to a variety of factors. To be diagnosed with high blood pressure, your blood pressure needs to be measured at several different visits to the doctor's office and at your home, too. Some people get so nervous in the doctor's office that their blood pressure is high there, but normal at home. Other things that can affect your blood pressure are:

- Exercise

- Stress

- Caffeine

- Tobacco

- Alcohol

- Time of day

When you check your blood pressure at home, keep these factors in mind. Try to be calm and well-rested for the most accurate test results.

Hypertension, Your Doctor, and You

If after a series of blood pressure readings you are diagnosed with hypertension, you will need to discuss a variety of issues with your doctor. A good doctor will want to know what you've been doing that may have caused your high blood pressure. This way, she can devise a plan of action based on your lifestyle that will help you get your blood pressure down and help you avoid more serious conditions like a heart attack or stroke. When you're talking with your doctor, be honest. Good doctors will not judge or reprimand you, they will want to help you. The best way for them to help is to have good, truthful information on how you live so they can offer sound advice.

The following paragraphs take you through some of the topics you and your doctor will discuss when you have high blood pressure.

What Medications Do You Take?

If you have high blood pressure, your doctor will ask what medications you are taking, even over-the-counter medications. Some over-the-counter medications, such as ibuprofen, cold and sinus remedies, and appetite suppressants, as well as some prescription drugs for depression, can raise your blood pressure. Your doctor will also ask you to stop smoking cigarettes, because they cause your blood vessels to constrict and raise blood pressure even more.

What Foods Do You Eat?

Your doctor will ask what foods you eat. Do you add salt to your food? Do you eat a lot of salty foods such as chips, canned soup, or processed meats? African Americans are more sensitive to salt, so too much salt—even what might be considered a normal amount—can raise your blood pressure. Drinking alcohol can raise your blood pressure, too.

Can you see where you might make changes to what you eat that will help bring your blood pressure down? Talk with your doctor about what foods to avoid or how to adjust what you eat now so it will have less impact on your blood pressure. Check out the DASH meal plan on page 138. By following it, you can bring your blood pressure down.

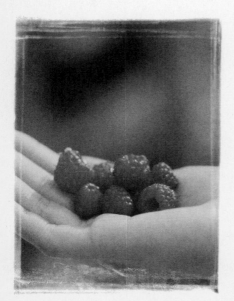

What about Exercise?

Your doctor will want to know how much exercise you do. I'm sure you already know that exercise can help lower your blood pressure. In fact, regular aerobic exercise is the best medicine for hypertension. Walking, jogging, swimming, bicycling, dancing, and rowing are all exercises that can help you. However, you should not lift heavy weights or do any heavy resistance exercises, which will raise your blood pressure and be hard on your heart. Lifting light weights should be okay, but get proper training to do it right.

As I mentioned in the last chapter, you may need an exercise stress test before you start an exercise program. Ask your doctor. The stress test can show how your heart operates during exercise, but don't just depend on the test. Listen to your body as you start exercising and build up slowly as you get stronger. Use your common sense. If your muscles are so sore you can barely move the next day, you overdid it. Go slow.

Weight Loss?

The doctor will ask whether you have gained or lost weight recently. Losing weight can help bring your blood pressure down. If your child is overweight and has high blood pressure, too, you will both benefit from eating less and making better food choices.

Diabetes?

If you also have diabetes, your doctor will ask more questions to determine whether you have nerve and blood vessel damage such as:

- Do you have numbness or tingling in your hands?

- Have you had any episodes of impotence?

- Have you had frequent urinary tract infections?

- Do you become dizzy when you stand up too quickly?

- Have you had a dilated eye exam recently? What were the results?

The Physical Exam

If it looks like you may have hypertension there are other things to check than just your blood pressure. Your doctor will examine your neck for extended veins, which could show heart failure. Heart failure happens when your heart cannot keep up with the excess demand on it. He will listen with a stethoscope on both sides of your windpipe for the sound of blood flowing through the neck arteries. He can hear if those arteries are narrowed and the blood supply to your brain is affected. He may check your eyes to see if there is any damage to the blood vessels on the retina at the back of your eye.

He will check to see if your heart is enlarged or if there is thickening of the heart wall due to the excess work that high blood pressure makes it do. The doctor will also listen to your lungs to see if there is any congestion, which goes along with heart failure. He'll listen to the arteries in your abdomen to check blood supply to your kidneys. He'll check for cysts in your kidneys, too.

What You Can Do

If you do have high blood pressure, it's not the end of the world. A lot of people react to hypertension by either dismissing it as not that important, or treating it like an irreversible omen of doom. Try to fall somewhere in the middle of this spectrum. Hypertension is too important to ignore, but it's also not a death certificate. There are things you can do.

If your blood pressure is not too high, you may be able to bring it down with lifestyle changes alone, such as stopping smoking and drinking alcohol, exercising more, and making better food choices. Losing five or ten pounds will help. There's research to back this up. A study called Trial of Mild Hypertension Study (TOMHS) showed that lifestyle changes alone lowered average blood pressure from 141/91 to 130/83 for 234 people after one year. What you do does have an effect on your blood pressure.

Generally, high blood pressure therapy fails because the person who has it doesn't make the lifestyle changes or doesn't take the prescribed medication. Sometimes this is because people don't understand what to do; sometimes the drugs cost too much. You have to decide whether you're willing to work to get your blood pressure down. You can do something about your condition. Use this power.

Lose Weight

If you are obese and have other health problems, such as diabetes, you will need medication to get your blood pressure down as quickly as possible. But medicine won't do everything. It is important to make the lifestyle changes, too. Change your eating habits. Try the DASH meal plan (see page 138). It is high in fiber and good fats, which help you feel full longer. You might try eating this way for a couple of months and see what effect it has on both your weight and your blood pressure. Then you may need less medication.

Blood Pressure Medications

The medications usually prescribed for high blood pressure are beta-blockers and diuretics. Diuretics are better known as water pills, and in low doses, they work well. They can cause potassium loss. If you take a diuretic and another drug to lower your blood pressure, watch out because it can drop very low. Beta-blockers (such as Inderal, Tenormin, and Lopressor) are used to treat angina (heart pain) and heart failure, because they lower blood pressure and heart rate. Beta-blockers can help prevent a second heart attack from occurring.

Another class of drugs used to treat high blood pressure are ACE inhibitors, which also slow down kidney disease. These are especially important drugs for people with diabetes. They do not affect blood glucose levels and don't raise your cholesterol levels, but they do have side effects. Your doctor must monitor your kidney function, and you may develop a cough, a common side effect.

Alpha-blockers also lower blood pressure, sometimes very deeply when you first begin taking them. They relax the blood vessels, don't affect blood glucose, and may have a good effect on cholesterol levels. You should take this drug at bedtime and rise slowly in the morning, to avoid dizziness. This drug also helps men with prostate enlargement and difficulty urinating.

Angiotensin II receptor blockers are very effective in lowering blood pressure. They reduce kidney damage, improve cholesterol levels, and don't have side effects like a cough. They are especially helpful in treating blood pressure and protecting kidney function in type 2 diabetes.

One of the side effects of blood-pressure medication that most concerns people is the effect on their sex life. Some of these drugs may cause impotence or a loss of sensation. Talk with your doctor about a lower dose or changing to a different drug. You may find this is the motivation to make some lifestyle changes now.

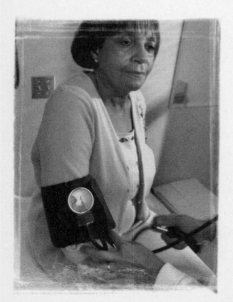

The DASH Eating Plan

The National Heart, Lung, and Blood Institute conducted two research studies, called the Dietary Approaches to

---

What Foods Are Good for Someone with High Blood Pressure?

- Vegetables and fruits and a little lean protein like fish and raw nuts—not salted ones.
- Unsalted food. Instead of layering everything with salt, expand your palate and try pepper, spices, lemon, lime, vinegar, or salt-free blends for flavor.
- Foods low on cheese or whole milk.
- Meals low in red meat. Daily burgers are not friendly to blood pressure. Remember that mustard, catsup, pickles, and sauces have salt in them, too.
- Frozen or fresh foods that don't come in a box or a can. While not all boxed and canned food is bad, much of it is crammed with trans fats and sodium. Read food labels to learn where sodium is hiding. It's hard to believe, but canned soup has four times as much salt as potato chips, even though the chips taste saltier. Neither one is good for high blood pressure.
- Unsalted water for cooking rice or pasta. Cut back on instant or flavored rice, pasta, and cereal mixes, which have added salt.

Stop Hypertension (DASH) studies, to see which food choices lower blood pressure. The first study showed that blood pressure came down when the participants ate meals that were heavy on fruits, vegetables, and low-fat dairy foods.

These meals were very low in saturated fat, cholesterol, and total fat. This eating plan—called the DASH meal plan—also included whole grains, fish, poultry, and nuts. What it did not have much of was red meat, sweets, or sugary beverages. It is rich in nutrients the body needs, such as magnesium, potassium, and calcium, as well as protein and fiber.

Who Was in the DASH Study?

There were actually two DASH studies. The first DASH study involved 459 adults with blood pressures measuring less than 160/95. One fourth of them had high blood pressure. Half were women, and more than half were African Americans. Two meal plans came out of this study as having the best effect on blood pressure.

The second DASH study looked at the effect of three different levels of sodium in these two meal plans. There were 412 participants. Half were women and a little more than half were African Americans, almost half of whom had high blood pressure. I told you we were prone to hypertension.

The Power of the DASH

Like I said, there were three different meal plans in the first DASH study. The first was a typical American diet; the second was the same meal plan plus lots of fruits and vegetables; and the third was the DASH eating plan. None of the meal plans were vegetarian or needed special foods. As you can imagine, the two that had a beneficial effect on blood pressure were the fruits and vegetables plan and the DASH plan, but the greatest effect came from the DASH plan. Plus, most people showed an improvement in blood pressure after only two weeks on the DASH meal plan.

The second DASH then took the two most effective meal plans (the fruits and vegetables plan and the DASH plan) and divided them into three different sodium levels—3,300 milligrams, 2,400 milligrams, and 1,500 milligrams a day. The DASH meal plan was more effective at lowering blood pressure than the American diet with more fruits and vegetables in it. The biggest drop in blood pressure happened in folks who were eating 1,500 mg of sodium on the DASH meal plan. The drop was most pronounced in folks with high blood pressure, but the other folks saw a drop in blood pressure, too.

The basic DASH eating plan is shown in Table 6-1. You can download a free, expanded copy or order one from the NHLBI Health Information Center using the contact information given at the end of this chapter. You can also get a free food journal, menus, and recipes.

As the DASH meal plan points out, most of the extra sodium in people's meals comes from processed foods. Look on the food label for reduced-sodium or no-salt-added products. Read the Nutrition Facts labels on everything, checking for the amount of sodium. There are Nutrition Facts labels on meats, too. Fresh meats, such as chicken and fish, have less salt than canned, smoked, or processed types.

Table 6-1. The DASH Meal Plan

The DASH eating plan shown below is based on 2,000 calories a day. The number of daily servings in a food group may vary from those listed, depending on your caloric needs. Use this chart to help you plan your menus or take it with you when you go to the store.

Food Group	Daily Servings (Except as Noted)	Serving Sizes	Examples and Notes	Significance of Each Food Group to the DASH Eating Plan
Grains and grain products	7–8	1 slice bread 1 oz dry cereal* 1/2 cup cooked rice, pasta, or cereal	Whole wheat bread, English muffin, pita bread, bagel, cereals, grits, oatmeal, crackers, unsalted pretzels and popcorn	Major sources of energy and fiber
Vegetables	4–5	1 cup raw leafy vegetable 1/2 cup cooked vegetable 6 oz vegetable juice	Tomatoes, potatoes, carrots, green peas, squash, broccoli, turnip greens, collards, kale, spinach, artichokes, green beans, lima beans, sweet potatoes	Rich sources of potassium, magnesium, and fiber
Fruits	4–5	6 oz fruit juice 1 medium fruit 1/4 cup dried fruit 1/2 cup fresh, frozen, or canned fruit	Apricots, bananas, dates, grapes, oranges, orange juice, grapefruit, grapefruit juice, mangoes, melons, peaches, pineapples, prunes, raisins, strawberries, tangerines	Important sources of potassium, magnesium, and fiber

Food Group	Servings	Serving Sizes	Examples	Significance
Low-fat or fat-free dairy foods	2–3	8 oz milk, 1 cup yogurt, 1 1/2 oz cheese	Fat-free (skim) or low-fat (1%) milk, fat-free or low-fat buttermilk, fat-free or low-fat regular or frozen yogurt, low-fat and fat-free cheese	Major sources of calcium and protein
Meats, poultry, and fish	2 or less	3 oz cooked meats, poultry, or fish	Select only lean; trim away visible fats; broil, roast, or boil instead of frying; remove skin from poultry	Rich sources of protein and magnesium
Nuts, seeds, and dry beans	4–5 per week	1/3 cup or 1/2 oz nuts, 2 Tbsp or 1/2 oz seeds, 1/2 cup cooked dry beans or peas	Almonds, filberts, mixed nuts, peanuts, walnuts, sunflower seeds, kidney beans, lentils	Rich sources of energy, magnesium, potassium, protein, and fiber
Fats and oils†	2–3	1 tsp soft margarine, 1 Tbsp lowfat mayonnaise, 2 Tbsp light salad dressing, 1 tsp vegetable oil	Soft margarine, low-fat mayonnaise, light salad dressing, vegetable oil (such as olive, corn, canola, or safflower)	DASH has 27 percent of calories as fat, including fat in or added to foods
Sweets	5 per week	1 Tbsp sugar, 1 Tbsp jelly or jam, 1/2 oz jelly beans, 8 oz lemonade	Maple syrup, sugar, jelly, jam, fruit-flavored gelatin, jelly beans, hard candy, fruit punch, sorbet, ices	Sweets should be low in fat

* Equals 1/2–1 1/4 cups, depending on cereal type. Check the product's Nutrition Facts Label.

† Fat content changes serving counts for fats and oils: For example, 1 Tbsp of regular salad dressing equals 1 serving; 1 Tbsp of a low-fat dressing equals 1/2 serving; 1 Tbsp of a fat free dressing equals 0 servings.

Adapted from *Facts About the DASH Eating Plan*, NHLBI Health Information Center, 2003.

Resources

Associations

The International Society on Hypertension in Blacks
2045 Manchester Street, NE
Atlanta, GA 30324
404-875-6263
www.ishib.org

The National Heart, Lung, and Blood Institute (NHLBI) of the National Institutes of Health (NIH) has an information center, where you can get free information about treatment, diagnosis, and prevention of heart, lung, and blood diseases.
NHLBI Health Information Center
P.O. Box 30105
Bethesda, MD 20824-0105
301-592-8573
TTY 240-629-3255
www.nhlbi.nih.gov

To hear recorded messages about high blood pressure prevention and treatment, call toll-free 800-575-9355. The information line also has messages on high cholesterol. The messages are available in English and Spanish.

7

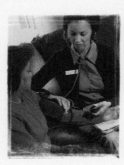

HEART DISEASE, STROKE, AND CHOLESTEROL

More than seven million Americans have coronary heart disease (CHD), a degenerative condition that severely affects the blood vessels of the heart and can lead to damaged heart muscle. It is the number one killer of Americans, far more prevalent than cancer and car accidents. But not only does it kill, it also affects a lot of living time by making people sick and miserable.

Your heart is the mighty pump that sends blood flowing throughout your body, picking up oxygen at your lungs and glucose in the intestines and carrying both to the cells, speeding the fighter white blood cells to injuries, and dropping wastes off at the kidneys and lungs. Your heart and blood vessels are the miracle network that makes your body go. It is absolutely necessary that you keep this system healthy.

Fortunately the heart is a muscle, and it responds well to exercise. In fact, runners tend to have a low pulse, meaning that their hearts beat very slowly. Their circulatory system is so healthy that it requires much less work to run smoothly at rest. It's good to get your heart used to changing rhythms, too. It needs your help to be strong, and to do its job well. By the food you feed it and the physical activity that you do, you either increase or damage the health of your heart and blood vessels. And this goes for children, too. As obesity and lack of exercise increase among the young, so does the risk of heart disease. A heart attack at the age of 24 used to be a tragic anomaly. Now it has become a distinct possibility. Do you want to see your children suffering heart attacks before you even reach middle age?

Are You at Risk?

Heart disease does not simply appear out of the blue one day. It is a gradual development that is marked by clear indications of an oncoming problem. If you are careful and work closely with your doctor, there is a good chance you can catch heart disease before it becomes fatal. You can then work to keep you and your heart healthy. First, you must know the risk factors and their signals.

Cholesterol and Blood Pressure— Early Warning System

Research and experience has shown us that there are two simple measures of the health of your heart and blood vessels. If you have high blood pressure or you have high blood cholesterol, your heart is in danger. You may feel fine, but the warning bell has rung. If you decide to take steps to lower your blood pressure and your cholesterol, you will do your heart—and yourself—the biggest favor possible.

Diabetes—A Heart Disease?

If you have diabetes, it's like you have already had your first heart attack. Yes, it's that bad. To stave off something fatally serious, you must develop a three-pronged goal:

1. Manage your diabetes for normal blood glucose
2. Lower your blood pressure
3. Lower your cholesterol levels

Fortunately the healthy lifestyle changes that improve one, improve them all.

The Emotional Heart

Recent research seems to be showing one other risk factor for heart disease—depression. It appeals to common sense, doesn't it, to think that a broken heart could lead to heart disease? Take care of depression. Go for counseling and learn healthy ways to cope with stress. You won't be surprised to find daily exercise and eating well on that list, will you? If you are taking antidepressants, tell your heart doctor, because they might cause problems with blood thinners or other heart medicines you may also be taking.

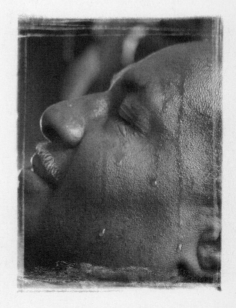

What Will a Heart Attack Feel Like?

You need to know the signs of a heart attack for yourself and others. During a heart attack it's important to get to the hospital immediately, so the doctors can

Table 7-1. Common Symptoms of Heart Attack

• Pain or tightness in your chest wall, jaw, back of neck, or down the left arm	• Nausea or vomiting
	• Sweating
• Shortness of breath	• Racing or skipping heart-beat or palpitations*
• Aching, throbbing, or squeezing sensation*	• Feeling like the heart jumps into the throat*
• Weakness, fatigue, or drowsiness*	• Blood sugar out of control
• Hot poker jab in the chest*	• Confusion

* These symptoms are most common to women.

try to save the heart from any more damage. Most everyone thinks that the sign of a heart attack is crushing chest pain, like an elephant sitting on your chest, but some people only have heavy sweating and nausea. Do not wait for the crushing pain. You may never get that symptom. Women often have different symptoms from men (Table 7-1. Common Symptoms of Heart Attack). People with nerve damage, from diabetes or alcoholism perhaps, may not feel chest pain either. Some people have only back pain or abdominal discomfort. Be alert to any of these symptoms. If you have diabetes, the sign of a heart attack may be something as subtle as out-of-control blood glucose levels.

The Clues Come from Cholesterol

The number one way to measure your chance of having a heart attack is to measure the amount of cholesterol in your blood. The second measure is your blood pressure (see Chapter 6). If both are high, you have work to do.

What Is Cholesterol?

Cholesterol is the name for the fats that travel around your body in the bloodstream. Your body uses fat to build cell walls and to make certain vitamins and hormones. Cholesterol and other fats:

- Form insulation around nerves

- Make bile, which is necessary for digesting fat and absorbing fat-soluble vitamins

- Serve as an important source of energy.

Your body uses triglycerides (another blood fat) for energy, to keep you warm, and to protect your organs. These blood fats, which are also called lipids, do not mix well with water and have to be carried by proteins so they can travel through the bloodstream. The fat and protein mixtures are called lipoproteins.

Based on the way they are put together and how much cholesterol is in them, lipoproteins can be divided into high-density lipoproteins (HDL), low-density lipoprotein (LDL), and triglycerides.

High-density lipoproteins (HDL) are made in the liver and contain little cholesterol. In fact, as they travel around in the bloodstream, they remove excess cholesterol and take it back to the liver to be broken down. That is why HDL is called the "good" cholesterol, and you want these levels as high as you can get them. Men want a level higher than 45 mg/dl and women want a level higher than 55 mg/dl. Exercise is the key.

Low-density lipoproteins (LDL) carry a lot of cholesterol from the liver throughout the body. This is the cholesterol that makes the buildup on the walls of arteries that leads to atherosclerosis. It is called "bad" cholesterol. LDL levels should be below 100 mg/dl. Food choices and weight have a strong effect on LDL levels.

Triglycerides are carried in the blood but are mostly stored in fat tissue. Your goal is probably 150 mg/dl or less.

Notice that each class of lipid is characterized by a certain number that represents the level that will reduce the risks for vascular disease (heart disease). Whenever your blood is tested for any of these (and for glucose), always get the number. Write it down. The only way to know how close you are to goal (or how much trouble you're in) is to *know the number*.

To provide you with more information about cholesterol, the NIH has set up the National Cholesterol Education Program (NCEP), which provides free advice and recipes, charts for your progress, a BMI calculator, a Virtual Fitness Room, and tips for how to read a food label. The contact information is listed in Resources at the end of this chapter.

High Cholesterol

When your doctor checks your cholesterol levels, he uses a blood test to measure your lipid levels. If your lipids are high, you have high cholesterol. That could mean that your total cholesterol is too high, or that your LDL (bad) cholesterol is too high and your HDL (good) cholesterol is too low. You see that your body needs to balance the bad cholesterol with the good.

High cholesterol is dangerous to your heart, because too much fat is traveling around in your blood. It is sticking to the sides of your blood vessels, narrowing them (which raises blood pressure), making them stiff and easier to damage. Narrow blood vessels are easier to block with a tiny blood clot or a piece of the lining of the blood vessel if it tears or breaks loose. This is what causes heart attacks and strokes.

What Can You Do to Improve Your Cholesterol?

Your risk of heart disease goes down six-fold the closer you get your HDL to 80. You may not be able to get your HDL level that high, but you can get closer than you are now. Any increase is beneficial. So, how do you do that? To raise your HDL (good) cholesterol:

- Exercise (this is *biggest* factor)

- Drink only one alcoholic beverage a day or less

- Stop smoking

- Lose weight

- Change your parents (just kidding. But the genes you inherited do play a large role)

- Take a cholesterol drug that lowers the bad and raises the good

Exercise Is the First Half

It's directly proportional. The more you exercise the higher your HDL. An Olympic athlete has the best HDL levels, a state-level athlete has the next best, a marathon runner has the next best, and so on. It's up to you how much you want to do. Every step does count where your heart is concerned.

Getting more exercise is great for lowering LDL as well as raising HDL.

Eating Well Is the Other Half

What diet lowers cholesterol? Your doctor may not know. You need meals with more fiber and less animal fats in them.

Research has shown that folks who eat a lot of fiber (25–35 grams of fiber a day) lower their LDL (bad) cholesterol. Whole grains, beans, vegetables, and fruits are the best sources of fiber. Oatmeal is advertised as a cholesterol-lowering food because it has soluble fiber. Steel cut oats have more fiber than "instant" oats.

Eat more beans. A favorite meal of my family has long been a pot of beans and cornbread. We buy stone ground corn meal and then refrigerate or freeze what we don't use. Grains that still have the germ and bran (the fiber and vitamins) in them can spoil. That's okay, because it's the natural, unprocessed foods with life in them that put life in you. Foods that can sit on a shelf for two or three years without even growing mold may not be the best choice. See Chapter 2 for more information about fiber and foods that contain it.

Eat more of the healthy fats that are found in nuts and fish. In fact, a handful or even two handfuls of almonds every day has been shown to have a strong benefit for your heart's health. Raw nuts are your best choice. Freeze them to keep the fat in them from going rancid. Roasted nuts are okay if they do not have vegetable oil or hydrogenated oil added. You'll have to read the food label to find out. Salted nuts won't do your blood pressure any good.

Here's something you may not know: Chocolate covered nuts also have good fats in the dark chocolate. An ounce of dark chocolate a day can be good for your heart. An ounce is a very little amount, though. Dark chocolate is better than milk chocolate, which has saturated fat from the milk. This tidbit of information may make you smile while you're making healthy food choices today. This doesn't mean it's healthy to have a candy bar every two hours. Too much sugar. A bit of chocolate is just another choice in a variety of foods. For example, ground up flax seed sprinkled in your cereal or cookies or casseroles gives you good fats, too.

Learn to be creative while you preserve the enjoyment of food. But always stay within the limits that will protect your health.

Back to the Mediterranean Diet

Research done on the healthy hearts of the people living in Greece, Italy, and France shows the benefit of eating the Mediterranean way—fresh foods, vegetables, fruit, olive oil, and lean meat or fish. This way of eating is now considered by Harvard University School of Public Health to be the way we can prevent heart disease.

We cannot overlook the fact that those folks in Greece, Italy, and France live at a more leisurely pace than we do, which takes a lot of stress out of the day. They also walk more and drive less than we do. They don't work so many hours, and they take longer, regular vacations. Vacation—which is often a month long—is scheduled into the year by government and businesses alike. Those are things to consider. Your company probably isn't going to spring for an extra month's vacation, but if you regularly unwind with yoga or deep breathing or take a trip to the park or the country to breathe fresh air and see green trees, you are dealing with your stress levels in healthy ways, too.

If you ask most people what they know about the Mediterranean diet, they remember only that a glass of wine or eating olive oil improves cholesterol levels. You need to eat all the foods, not just one or two. You need to invest in the whole package to get the heart protection and benefits.

What about Medicine for Cholesterol?

If the medicine of food and exercise is not enough to get your cholesterol levels where they need to be for your health, then your doctor will recommend medication. Statin drugs really work. The HDL Atherosclerosis Treatment Study (HATS), a 3-year trial, compared the effect of niacin (a drug that raises HDL levels but may also raise blood glucose levels) and of statin on cholesterol levels. The statin group had these results:

- LDL (bad)   1/3 drop
- TG (triglycerides) 1/3 drop
- HDL (good)   1/3 rise

Talk with your doctor about which cholesterol-lowering drug might work best for you.

An Aspirin a Day . . .

Most scientists and doctors are agreed that there is a clear benefit to your heart from taking an aspirin every day. This is a preventive step. If you are already taking a blood thinner, like Coumadin, you may not need the blood-thinning action

---

Another Doctor's Advice

John LaPuma is an internist, professional chef, and former cooking school teacher. He runs the Santa Barbara Institute for Medical Nutrition and Healthy Weight. His suggestions for heart-healthy food choices are simple:

- Try leaving out red meat and dairy fats, such as cheese or whole milk.
- Try whole-wheat pasta instead of white flour pasta.
- Try unrefined barley in your soup instead of pearl barley that has had the outer layer, with its healthy ingredients, polished away.
- Use whole-wheat pita bread instead of regular bread, because it can hold all those wonderful vegetables you seek to eat.

Steps to take to prevent heart disease	
• Take a baby aspirin every day	• Get daily exercise
• Lower cholesterol levels	• Lose weight
• Stop smoking	• Lower blood pressure
• Eat more fruits and vegetables	• Reduce stress

of the aspirin, too. Ask your doctor if you should take an aspirin a day, because it may be your first step toward better heart health.

Stroke

The combination of cholesterol damage to blood vessels and high blood pressure that causes heart attacks can cause strokes, too. A stroke happens when something interferes with the blood supply to the brain. If the brain has to go without oxygen, parts of it can be damaged. You prevent a stroke and keep your brain healthy in the same ways that you protect your heart, too.

For unknown reasons African American males, even young boys, are more likely to have strokes than other groups of males. Many people have short-lasting symptoms that are like having a stroke (see the box "Warning Signs of a Stroke"). These events are called transient ischemic attacks (TIAs). These are serious signals from your body that a stroke is on the way. See a doctor now.

The benefits that you gain from good food and daily exercise are shared with your brain and help protect you against having a stroke, too.

Women and Heart Disease

It's not a guy thing. One in every three women dies of a heart attack. If you are over 50 years old, have diabetes, and you

Warning Signs of Stroke

- Sudden weakness or numbness of the face, arm, or leg on one side of the body
- Sudden dimness or loss of vision, particularly in one eye
- Loss of speech or trouble talking or understanding speech or writing
- Unexplained dizziness, unsteadiness when walking, or sudden falls
- Sudden, severe headaches with no obvious cause

are overweight, your chances of having a heart attack are very high.

If you are a woman, your symptoms of a heart attack are very likely to be different from the ones that men have. You may be expecting a pain in your left arm and shoulder and your chest. But many women never have that symptom. Some women feel nauseated and weak. Some may sweat and feel a dull ache in their back. You need to know what symptoms are more common in women and look out for them, too.

Estrogen, a hormone produced by the body, gives women an advantage against heart disease, but you lose that protection at menopause. If you have diabetes, you have lost that protection, too. You are four times more likely to have a heart attack if you have diabetes.

One way to protect your heart and keep it well is to not smoke, or to quit smoking right away. A recent and ongoing study of health information obtained from thousands of female nurses collected over a long period of time has shown this clearly. One part of the study focused on women with type 2 diabetes. Those nurses who smoked were more than twice as likely to have heart disease as nurses who never smoked or who had stopped smoking. Those women who smoked more than 15 cigarettes a day were eight times more likely to suffer from heart disease and stroke. The study proved that quitting smoking helps cut your risk. After 10 years, those who had quit smoking had the same health outlook as those who had never smoked at all.

The Kids Can Get It, Too

Let Us Start Preventing Their Heart Disease Now

Our children are now at risk for developing heart disease early in their lives and dying very young because they are too obese. Pretty much all we doctors can do is check their weight, blood pressure, and cholesterol levels and recommend ways to get these levels where they need to be. The rest is up to you and your child. It is much more important to stress lifestyle changes with your children, since the medication used to treat these problems are not generally approved for children. You know what to do to lower blood pressure and cholesterol for yourself, so you know what to do for your child, too. If your child is above the 85th percentile on a height/weight chart for his age, he and his heart are in the danger zone. You need to take action now.

You can talk with your child about the healthy changes that the family is going to take. Some example actions the family can take include:

- Not drinking so much soda at home or when you are out.

- Cooking more at home and not eating fast food every night or for lunch every day.

- Packing lunches for the next day every evening with your children.

- Keeping the morning peaceful so you can all enjoy breakfast together.

What Mom and Dad Must Help Their Kids Do:

- Limit TV and computer time to two hours a day
- Take a 30- to 45-minute walk every day
- Not smoke
- Eat more fruits and vegetables
- Eat less sat fat and trans fat (fast foods and processed foods)
- Eat less sugar

Try to make healthy foods available to your children. Don't bring home processed and fast foods, like pizza and fried chicken on a regular basis. If they always choose candy bars and colas for a snack, then don't bring those home either. These items should be viewed as special treats for special occasions. Offer them popcorn (popped fat-free in a hot-air popper). It tastes great and the fiber makes you feel pleasantly full. None of us wants to feel hungry 30 minutes after we eat. You can also help them take these extra little steps:

- Eat fruit for a snack instead of chips or cookies.

- Check the food label on the cereal box. Find ones with less sugar in them.

- Cook oatmeal with nuts and raisins for breakfast (your own, not instant with more sugar than you want).

- Fast food hamburger and hot dog buns have sugar in them, too. Plus they are made of white flour, which has had the healthy parts—the wheat germ and the bran (fiber)—removed. You can skip eating the bun, or make your own burgers at home with whole-wheat buns.

Each member of your family can make a difference in your own lives. Be proud of what you are doing. This is real, and this is important to you.

Make This the Land of Healthy Hearts

If we all pitch in and help each other, we can do away with heart disease as the number one killer in America. The little choices you make in what to eat and whether to walk for another 10 minutes today may not seem very important, but they add up to something that you can't buy and no one else can give you—your good health. Beyond that, your quiet, steady example can change everyone around you—and keep their hearts beating in healthy harmony. What a gift you give by the choices you make.

Resources

Associations

American Heart Association
National Center
7272 Greenville Avenue
Dallas, TX 75231
800-242-8721
www.americanheart.org

The American Diabetes Association
The ADA has a program called Make the Link. Web-based
animation explains the link between diabetes and heart disease. It defines diabetes, gives the ABCs, and tips for healthy
eating, exercise, and medications.
www.diabetes.org/MaketheLink

American Stroke Association
A Division of the American Heart Association
7272 Greenville Avenue
Dallas, TX 75231
888-478-7653
www.strokeassociation.org

Cardiovascular Health Program
Centers for Disease Control and Prevention
Mail Stop K-13
4770 Buford Highway, NE
Atlanta, GA 30341-3717
770-488-5080
www.cdc.gov/cvh

National Cholesterol Education Program
National Heart, Lung, and Blood Institute Health
Information Center
P.O. Box 30105
Bethesda, MD 30105

301-592-8573
www.nhlbi.nih.gov

Offers Heart Healthy Home Cooking: African American
Style, 20 recipes, $3.00.

National Diabetes Education Program (NDEP)
1 Diabetes Way
Bethesda, MD 20892-3600
800-438-5383
www.ndep.nih.gov

Books

Keeping Your Heart Healthy Despite Diabetes, by Marie
McCarren. American Diabetes Association, 2002.

CHAPTER

8

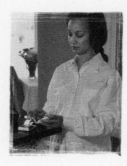

DIABETES

A Touch of Sugar?

Diabetes in the United States has reached almost epidemic proportions. As we grow bigger in the belly and less active—two of the main causes of type 2 diabetes—the condition blossoms. Plus, with fast food and modern convenience spreading around the globe, this epidemic is fast becoming a worldwide phenomena.

So what can we do? Not surprisingly, the very same things we do to keep our heart healthy and prevent other conditions—eat right and exercise. Unfortunately, most people don't focus on prevention. They wait until the disease strikes and then begin to focus on their health. Hopefully you'll be on the prevention team, but if not, don't worry—there are many successful methods to manage your diabetes. Before we get into specifics, though, we should probably discuss what exactly diabetes is.

What Is Diabetes?

Diabetes is the occurrence of high blood sugar as the result of a malfunction in the metabolism of food that happens because the pancreas stops making the hormone insulin or doesn't make enough. Insulin helps your body use the fuel it takes in from food. When you eat, the food is changed in your stomach and intestines into a sugar called glucose. Glucose then enters your bloodstream from the intestines. Then it waits for insulin to show up and open the doors to the cells, so it can get inside and provide energy for your body.

If there is no insulin, or not enough, glucose just hangs around in your bloodstream, waiting. Your cells are still hungry and you're not getting any of the fuel you ate for energy. So you eat more food, and that glucose enters the blood and stays there, too. Pretty soon you have high levels of glucose in your blood. This is bad because blood glucose (BG), or blood sugar as most folks call it, is a sticky substance. When you have high blood sugar day after day for years, it damages blood vessels and nerves all over the body. This is how high blood sugar causes the complications of diabetes in body parts such as eyes, feet, kidneys, and heart.

You can help glucose move into the cells with exercise. Exercise makes the muscles in your body pull glucose straight from the bloodstream. Plus, the more in shape you are, the better your insulin works for opening the doors to your cells. You can help it with diabetes pills or injections of insulin. These medications tell the body to produce more insulin, or to use the insulin that is already there better. Injections provide more insulin for the body to use.

Some people with type 2 diabetes find that better food choices and exercise are enough to get the blood sugar level down to normal. Some people need to take one or several kinds of diabetes pills. Some people need insulin to get the levels back where they belong. The good news is that we have all these ways to get energy into the cells and to lower your glucose level. This keeps you healthy.

Are There Different Types of Diabetes?

There are three main types of diabetes:

- Type 1 diabetes
- Type 2 diabetes
- Gestational diabetes

Type 1 diabetes. Type 1 diabetes is an autoimmune disorder where the body's immune system, for reasons still unknown, attacks the insulin-making cells of the pancreas (also known as the beta cells). The result is that the pancreas can no longer make insulin. People who have type 1 diabetes must have insulin injections to stay alive. Usually type 1 diabetes develops in younger people, sometimes even newborn babies.

About 1 million people have type 1 diabetes in the United States. African Americans are not necessarily more prone to this type of diabetes than other populations. So far, we don't have a way to prevent it or cure it. We can manage it very well, especially with the help of new insulins, new injection devices, blood glucose meters, and insulin pumps.

Type 2 diabetes. Type 2 diabetes is much more common than type 1—about 16 million people in the United States have it. African Americans are twice as likely to have it. Type 2 diabetes is different than type 1 in that the pancreas still makes insulin. It's just that for some reason, either the pancreas doesn't make enough or the body doesn't use the insulin well. Whatever the reason, blood sugar is high.

Not being able to use the insulin your body makes is called insulin resistance, which usually occurs in grown-ups and children who are thick in the middle. In response to low insulin use, the pancreas pumps out more insulin to get the glucose out of the blood. But the body can't use the insulin, so it travels around in the bloodstream, too. This cycle of low efficiency and overworked organs can't last forever. Eventually, the beta cells in the pancreas are going to wear out.

We do know how to prevent type 2 diabetes in people at high risk, as several large, well-designed scientific studies have shown. We have that secret for you. To prevent diabetes you need to exercise, eat right, and lose a little weight—losing 10 to 15 pounds makes a big difference. If you already have type 2 diabetes, these same steps help you bring your blood sugar back to normal, too.

Gestational Diabetes. This form of diabetes occurs during the stress of pregnancy. The hormones of pregnancy cause insulin resistance in the mother's body, so she has higher than normal blood sugar levels. This can be dangerous for the baby and for the mother. The baby is often very large from the excess insulin stimulated by the high amounts of glucose traveling around in the mother's blood.

Sometimes the mother can manage her blood sugar with exercise and planned menus. Sometimes she needs insulin to help her bring those blood sugar levels down. After the baby is born, the insulin resistance and diabetes go away. But about half of the women who have gestational diabetes will develop type 2 later in life.

What Other Factors Contribute to Diabetes?

First, you have to have the genes for diabetes. Many African Americans do. Type 2 diabetes generally runs in the family. If you have a family member with diabetes, you probably have the gene. But even if no one in your family has diabetes, you might still have inherited the gene.

In addition to a genetic predisposition, then there has to be a trigger that sets the genes off. For some people the trigger is a serious stress, like a car accident and surgery or the stress of pregnancy. For many people, the trigger is obesity. In fact, a lifestyle of sitting and eating too much seems to set the stage for the genes to express effects, especially in our children.

There are a lot of things about diabetes that, despite what a lot of people say and believe, are not true. For example, eating sugar does not cause diabetes. Also, it is okay to eat sugar when you have diabetes because it is just another carbohydrate (carb) to your body. All carbohydrates are turned into glucose, making up the "sugar" in your blood. The sugar you are eating is a little different from the glucose in your blood. But remember that your body prefers the carbohydrate from fruits, vegetables, and whole grains for the nutrients in them, but sugar is okay from time to time.

Who Gets Diabetes?

Diabetes is becoming an epidemic around the world. One of the reasons is that in every country, people have moved from the farm where they did heavy physical work for many hours each day to the city where they sit too much and eat too much food, especially fatty foods.

In the United States, 17 million people have been diagnosed with diabetes, and almost 16 million more are in the "pre-diabetes" stage. Pre-diabetes means your blood sugars are higher than normal but not at diabetes levels yet. This category was set up so people could start taking better care of themselves sooner. About half the people with pre-diabetes go on to develop type 2 diabetes within 10 years. But just because glucose levels aren't at diabetes levels doesn't mean that damage isn't being done. High blood sugar damages the body in pre-diabetes, too.

Almost three million African Americans have diabetes right now, but nearly a third of them don't know it. That may be why we suffer from twice as much diabetes-related blindness and lower leg amputations. We can't manage a condition that we don't know we have.

The fact is that one in every four African Americans between the ages of 65 and 75 has diabetes. One in every four African American women aged 55 or older has diabetes. The odds are high that diabetes is happening to someone near and probably very dear to you. Our rate of diabetes has tripled in the past 30 years, and the number continues to rise. A rise of this magnitude over so short a period of time indicates that it is the result of choices we have made in our lifestyles and not because our genes have changed. Our genes have not changed for many thousands of years, but clearly our *jeans* are changing much too fast—they're getting bigger and bigger! We need to make healthier choices to put the brakes on the twin epidemics of obesity and diabetes.

Type 2 diabetes is also on the rise among our children. One in three African American children will develop diabetes in his or her lifetime—and the way things are going that may be before they reach adulthood.

These are serious facts. Clearly it is time for us to become experts on this disease. First you have to know if you have it (see the box "Do You [or Someone You Love] Have Diabetes?"). You have to know if your child has it. Then you need to do everything you can to manage it so your blood sugar levels are close to normal. That's how you and your children can stay healthy.

What Are the Symptoms of Diabetes?

This depends on what type of diabetes it is. The symptoms of type 1 diabetes are generally more acute than those of type 2 and set in almost immediately. Type 2 diabetes is a little more gradual. You don't feel different when you first get type 2 diabetes. Nothing hurts to warn you of the seriousness of this

Do You (or Someone You Love) Have Diabetes?

The answers to these questions can show your chances of having diabetes. Circle the points under yes for statements that are true for you. If a statement is not true, circle zero. Add the points to get your total score.

Could You Have Diabetes?	Yes	No
I had a baby weighing more than 9 pounds at birth.	1 point	0
I have a sister or brother with diabetes.	1 point	0
I have a parent with diabetes.	1 point	0
My weight is the same or more than that listed in the weight chart below.	5 points	0
I am under 65 years of age *and* I get little or no exercise.	5 points	0
I am between 45 and 64 years of age.	5 points	0
I am 65 years of age or older.	9 points	0

If you score 10 points or more: Your risk is high for having diabetes. Only your health care provider can check to see if you have diabetes. Go find out. You need to know.

If your score is 3 to 9 points: Your risk for diabetes appears to be low now. But don't forget about it (especially if you are Hispanic/Latino, African American, American Indian, Asian American, or a Pacific Islander. Your risk may be higher in the future.

In the meantime, you can keep your risk low by losing weight if you are overweight, being physically active most days of the week, and eating meals that are high in fruits, vegetables, and whole grain foods. And don't forget the healthy fats.

Do You (or Someone You Love) Have Diabetes? (*continued*)

At-Risk Weight Chart

Height (feet/inches without shoes)	Weight (pounds without clothes)
4'10"	129
4'11"	133
5'0"	138
5'1"	143
5'2"	147
5'3"	152
5'4"	157
5'5"	162
5'6"	167
5'7"	172
5'8"	177
5'9"	182
5'10"	188
5'11"	193
6'0"	199
6'1"	204
6'2"	210
6'3"	216
6'4"	221

If you weigh the same or more than the amount listed for your height, you may be at risk for diabetes. Check with your doctor about your child's weight. Generally children at the 85 percentile in weight/height for their age group are at risk.

disease. Nothing hurts for years. But just because you don't hurt does not mean diabetes is not hurting you. Your blood sugars get higher, so you feel sluggish and weary. You get irritable and cranky. Your vision blurs, but it's such a gradual change that you don't realize what is happening. You start wearing glasses or keep getting new prescriptions. You're tired all the time, and you can't remember the last time you felt really good. The folks around you 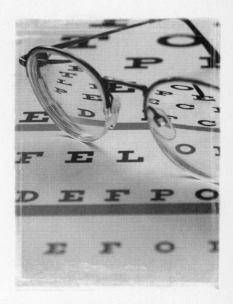 can't either. Your feet and toes might burn, which you notice at night, as the nerves are affected by high blood sugar.

The symptoms of diabetes are actually the symptoms of high blood sugar. These include:

- Blurry vision

- Headache

- Frequent urination

- Great thirst

- Hunger

- Weight loss without trying

- Tingling hands and feet

If you or other members of your family have diabetes, watch your children for signs of high blood sugar. Diabetes moves faster in children and you don't want them to end up in the emergency room. Know the symptoms of high blood sugar and keep an eye out for them. If your children combine the genes for diabetes with the triggers of obesity and no exercise, they are just waiting for the diagnosis.

Type 2 Diabetes Is Not a Kid's Disease

And Yet . . .

Our children are getting it. Type 2 diabetes in children occurs almost exclusively in African American and Latino children. Puberty is a time of raging hormones, which causes insulin resistance. Even kids without diabetes have 30% higher insulin levels during puberty. Add to this a lifestyle of too much processed food and no exercise, and you find weight gain and type 2 diabetes.

We don't want our children to have type 2 diabetes because then they can get all the grown-up complications of diabetes: heart attacks, stroke, kidney disease, eye disease, and nerve damage. These complications start showing up when the kids are in their twenties. This is wrong. A child diagnosed at the age of 20 can expect to lose 17 years of life to the disease.

Exercise slam dunks everything else when it comes to preventing diabetes. Wear a pedometer and aim for walking

---

You Can Prevent Type 2 Diabetes in Yourself and in Your Children

1. Exercise. If you walk for 150 minutes a week (30 minutes a day for 5 days of the week), you reduce your risk of getting diabetes by 58 to 70%. Now, that's power.

2. Eat right. Give your body premium fuel, especially five or more servings of fruits and veggies every day.

3. Lose weight if you need to. Then your body needs less insulin to do the job. If you do the first two steps, this one usually happens on its own.

10,000 steps a day. Yes, it's that simple. Buy one for your kids. It's a toy that can save their lives. Your challenge is to get more steps into the day (see Chapter 3). Being more active every day makes a huge difference in preventing type 2 diabetes.

Put your focus on wellness, not illness. When the whole family is involved in making healthy lifestyle choices, the children are much more likely to be active, choose better foods, lose weight, and get their diabetes under control. They learn the tools from their parents, who learn by teaching what they most need to know. We can all help each other be well. Read about Program ENERGY on page 264.

When You Are Diagnosed

When an adult gets diagnosed with type 2 diabetes, you have probably already had it 5 years or more. It's the symptoms of a diabetes complication that usually bring people to the doctor. You cannot feel what diabetes is doing until late in the game. That's why you want to catch it early, when you can do something to head it in a healthy direction.

See your doctor at least two to four times a year because you need help managing this disease. In fact, you are going to need the help of your doctor, nurse educator, dietitian, dentist, ophthalmologist, and other health specialists to help you manage diabetes and stay healthy. Regular visits to see how you are doing are important to your success. What you choose to eat and to do for exercise every day are the most important decisions of all. Dietitians and fitness trainers can help you succeed with a new lifestyle.

Why Don't People Take Care of Themselves?

Many people have what I call "deniabetes." They don't want the disease, so they ignore it or expect the doctor to take care of it. Your doctor does not have your diabetes. You have your diabetes. It is your daily challenge. If all you know about diabetes is what you've heard from family members or friends, then you don't know enough about diabetes. The scary stories about amputations and kidney failure do not have to come true in your life. We have the tools now and the knowledge to take much better care of diabetes than people had even 10 years ago. However, the tools are no good if you don't use them.

The research results are clear: Keeping your blood sugar levels normal or near normal can keep you healthy. The Diabetes Control and Complications Trial (DCCT) studied nearly 1,500 people with type 1 diabetes for nearly 10 years. The study was ended early to tell people with diabetes that managing blood sugar to normal levels prevented most complications from even developing and slowed down others. This puts the power back in your hands and dispels the doom. The same benefits of managing your blood sugar levels for people with type 2 diabetes were seen in a large study called the United Kingdom Prospective Diabetes Study (UKPDS). In all the research, there is no question about the results. Taking care of your diabetes today gives you more and better tomorrows. By reaching the treatment goals that include an A1C (a number that indicates your glucose level over a three-month period. See below) of less than 7%, improved lipids, and more normal blood pressure, you can get a 60 to 70% chance of not even developing a complication. If you already have a complication, you can slow it down, and in some cases, reverse the damage. If I had odds like these on the lottery, I would buy a ticket every day because I would win four or five days of the week. Taking care of your diabetes is definitely worth the time it takes.

Managing Diabetes

To manage diabetes you need to know what your blood sugars are. Use a glucose meter, check your blood sugar often, and get a notebook and keep a thorough record of everything. You need to know what to improve before you can improve it.

Next, know what makes your blood sugar go up and what makes it go down. Food raises blood sugar. Exercise and medication lower it. It seems simple, and theoretically it is. But usually things aren't this cut and dry. Other things can get into the mix. Some days you won't be able to figure out what made your blood sugar so high or so low. Talk over your records with your health care team, and don't despair if some numbers are a mystery. There will always be a few that even Sherlock Holmes couldn't figure out. Don't get too upset about the occasional number that is out of line. Remember, it's the long-term or average exposure that your body will show the greatest responses to.

Think of the numbers on your blood glucose meter as you do the gas gauge in your car. The number helps you decide whether to refuel because the number is low or to go for a walk because it's high. In your notebook record your blood glucose numbers and what time you check, how much carbohydrate you eat at each meal, how much exercise you do, when you are sick or under stress, and when you take your medications. Check the lists below for things to note in your record. This can help you remember to take your medication each day, and you can see how many carbs you usually eat at each meal (see Chapter 2).

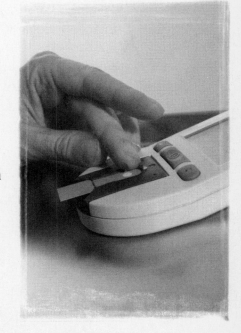

Good records give you the information you need to be able to see the patterns of your day, which helps you manage your blood sugar levels. Try to find trends and work with your health care team to figure out what might be causing these trends.

These raise blood sugar:	These lower blood sugar:
Food, especially carbohydrate	Insulin and diabetes pills
	Exercise
Illness or infection	Laughter
Worrying	Deep breathing and slow
Anger	stretches
Growth spurts	School exams or thinking
Hormones	hard
Injury (BG spikes, then falls)	Cold
Getting mad in traffic	

Run experiments to find out how much different things affect your blood glucose. Eat a food, such as two slices of pizza, and then two hours later, check your blood glucose. How high did the carb in the pizza make your blood glucose go? To see the power of exercise, you can check your blood glucose, take a 45-minute walk, and check your blood again about 30 minutes later. How much did the exercise lower your blood sugar level? You have a tool to see what works for your body. It is your blood glucose meter. Usually the target ranges for blood sugar are 80–120 mg/dl before meals and below 160 mg/dl after meals. Ask your doctor what your target ranges are.

Why Check Your Blood Sugar?

You get some really important information from that little meter. In a study of the people who use their blood sugar meters every day, seven out of ten had an A1C (see the section below) less than 8. Of another group who just used their meters a couple of times a month, only two people in ten had

High Blood Sugar (Hyperglycemia) Can Happen if You:	Low Blood Sugar (Hypoglycemia) Can Happen if You:
• Eat too much • Are sick or under stress • Do not exercise • Do not take your insulin or diabetes pills	• Skip a meal or snack • Don't eat all your meal or snack • Don't eat at the right time • Exercise more than usual • Drink too much alcohol • Take too much insulin or too many pills

an A1C less than 8. There's a clear health benefit to the folks who use their BG meters often.

So, Why Don't People Check Their BG More Often?

• **Reason 1—It hurts**. Check with your nurse educator about the latest diabetes equipment and to be sure you are getting a blood sample correctly. Your hands should be clean and *dry*. You don't need to clean the site with alcohol, but if you do, be sure that it is dry before you use the lancet. Use the sides of your fingers, not the pad in the middle. New meters take blood from less painful sites, such as your forearm or thigh, though these tests can be less accurate. You'll need to know when it's okay to use alternative sites and when you'll need to prick your finger to test.

• **Reason 2—Forget to take the meter to work or school.** Can you afford to have two meters—one for home and one for work? This may help. Or, set up a kit or backpack with all you need to check your blood and carry it with you everywhere.

- **Reason 3—Test strips cost too much.** You might be able to cut the strips in two lengthwise, so you have two for the price of one. Otherwise, once you have set up your meal plan and exercise habits, you may not have to check as often. When you count the carbohydrate in your meals, and eat about the same amount of carb at the same meals from day to day, your BG should fall into a pattern. Getting your diabetes under control means you can check less.

Ask your doctor or diabetes educator when to check. They can help you set up a schedule over two weeks that will give you enough information to find patterns but that won't make you check before and after every meal. They may be able to work with your insurance company to get you more strips. Fasting glucose (the one you check first thing in the morning) is probably most important if you just check once a day.

What Is an A1C Test and Why Do I Need One?

An A1C test is a blood test that is usually done in the doctor's office. Your A1C is your blood-sugar "batting average" over the past two to three months. It includes all the highs and lows and gives you the average glucose level for two months. Not eating before you take the test won't make any difference to the results. If you have an A1C test done at least every six months, you can see how well you are managing your blood sugar levels. People with type 1 diabetes or with problems controlling their blood sugar levels may have an A1C every three months. The target A1C for most people with diabetes is less than 7. Managing your glucose over the long run is very important. The power of the UKPDS was the one-two punch of tight blood pressure control and an A1C of 6.8.

Type 2 Management: Exercise, Meal Planning, Oral Meds, Insulin

Nothing is more important to managing type 2 diabetes than your meals and your exercise. These are the foundation for anything else you do to treat this disease. These two treatments may be enough to lower your morning (fasting) blood glucose and your after-meal blood glucose to normal levels. Or you may need to take a diabetes pill. Or you may need to take two different diabetes pills. Or you may need a pill and insulin injections. The medications can help you reach your daily blood glucose goals and your A1C goal.

Please don't let anything stop you from using insulin if you need to. Don't wait until your A1C is 10 or higher. An A1C of 10 means that your treatment isn't working for you and you need to make some changes now. The chart below can help you see what the changes might be. You may do fine with diet and exercise for a few years, but then all of a sudden your next A1C is a 9. This may mean your body is not making as much insulin. Your doctor can prescribe a diabetes medication to help bring your A1C back down to 7 over the next three months.

A1C Level	Treatment
Less than or equal to 7	Diet and exercise
Less than or equal to 8	1 type of diabetes pill
Less than or equal to 9	2 or more types of pills
Less than or equal to 10	Insulin

Unfortunately, this usually works in a pattern of stages just like this. We need to avoid this pattern. When your A1C gets higher than 7 and remains that way, it is time to change treatment. The mistake we make is waiting too long to be more aggressive in our treatment. The aim is to get to goal and stay there!

The ABCs of Being Healthy with Diabetes

Diabetes puts you at a much higher risk for heart attack and stroke. It's often said that having diabetes is like already having your first heart attack. That's why the ABCs of diabetes are: A1C, Blood pressure, and Cholesterol. The goals for most people are:

A1C	less than 7
Blood pressure	120/80
Cholesterol	LDL: under 100 mg/dl
	HDL: over 45 mg/dl for men; over 55 mg/dl for women
	Triglycerides: under 150 mg/dl

To get to your goals you may need to take an ACE inhibitor and a daily aspirin, but once you're there, you've cut your chance of getting heart disease, kidney failure, and eye disease by more than half. You can't get a higher return on your investment of time and money than that.

Diet and exercise never fail you. They are always your number one defense and offense against disease. But eventually they may not be enough to keep your A1C down. The disease progresses. Keep doing what you need to do to keep your A1C in the healthiest range. A healthy lifestyle always helps you more than drugs can, and it helps the drugs work better.

It's a Family Affair

Diabetes is striking the whole family. It's time to bring the family in and talk about what is going on. It's time to involve the family in planning meals, shopping for meals, working in the garden, and cooking meals together. Teenagers make excellent chefs. They just need some encouragement and success. Homemade food is better than any other food. Dine in together instead of eating out so often. Be home and be well together.

If you get involved with your children's health, especially if they already have diabetes, research shows that these children get much better A1C levels (7) than kids whose families do not support them at all (12). You do not want your child's A1C in the double-digit range. High A1Cs show that she is in real danger. Do something!

Treatment for Type 2 in Kids

Most kids with type 2 diabetes see pediatric endocrinologists. These doctors are used to seeing kids with type 1 diabetes and accustomed to prescribing insulin. Insulin works for kids with type 2 as well, but if you help your child change the way she eats and exercise regularly, her blood sugar levels will come down, and she may not need any more insulin or diabetes pills to control her blood sugar levels. Lifestyle makes such a difference to our children.

Take Action
Knowing that diabetes may live at your house means nothing if you don't do anything about it. Find out if you or your children have it. Get the blood test. Watch for the symptoms. Together enjoy daily exercise, and eat more vegetables, too.

Type 1 Diabetes

People with type 1 diabetes must take insulin to live. We have found that the best way to do this is to try to copy the way the pancreas releases insulin when we eat and at other

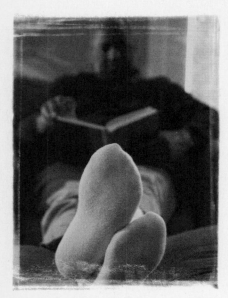

times during the day. To do this you need four or more injections a day. You need to check your blood glucose even more often to decide how much insulin to take and when.

Rapid-acting insulin brings down the blood sugar rise after each meal, and long-acting insulin assists in other bodily processes. Multiple daily injections is one way to copy the body's release of insulin during the day and night. Using an insulin pump to release a tiny bit of background insulin each hour and more insulin to match the carbohydrate eaten at a meal is another way to mimic the body. Both methods give you much more control over the rise and fall of your blood sugar levels than ever before.

Clearly your blood glucose meter is your best friend and needs to go everywhere with you, and the A1C is an important measure of how well you are balancing your blood sugars every day.

Your Feet Have Carried You All the Way

No matter whether you have type 1 or type 2 diabetes, damage to your nerves can leave your feet numb. If your feet are numb, you can't feel a piece of glass when you step on it. Some people have walked around for weeks with something sticking into their foot without knowing it. Such an injury can easily get infected and can cause real problems for you. Even when you take antibiotics, poor circulation makes healing take longer. Your immune system has to travel through the bloodstream, too.

That is why you want to check your feet every day. Look at the tops and bottoms. Feel them with your hands to see if there are swollen or hot spots from an infection. Check your shoes to be sure that there are no stones or tacks in them. Wear cushioned socks without thick toe seams. Choose well-fitting walking or running shoes with support for your feet and don't ever go barefoot.

These are pretty simple steps to follow for an outcome that is simply staggering. By merely doing a routine foot exam, it has been shown that as much as 50% of the foot amputations in diabetes can be prevented.

Low Blood Sugar

If you take insulin or certain diabetes pills, such as the sulfonylureas, your blood sugar can get too low (hypoglycemia), and you may pass out. Ask your doctor if your diabetes medication can cause this to happen. You need to know your own symptoms of low blood sugar, and to tell your family, friends, and co-workers what your symptoms are, so they can help you. If your blood sugar level is too low, you will not be able to help yourself (see the box "Symptoms of Low Blood Sugar").

Symptoms of Low Blood Sugar	
• Clumsiness	• Nervousness
• Confusion	• Numbness
• Fatigue	• Pounding heart
• Headache	• Sleepiness
• Stomachache	• Stubbornness
• Shakiness	• Sweating
• Feeling faint or empty	• Weakness
• Feeling upset or angry	• Light-headedness
• Nausea	

When your blood sugar is too low, you need some carbohydrate fast. If you can chew, eating some jelly beans or drinking a cup of low-fat milk or fruit juice can raise your blood sugar quickly. If you are not conscious, your helper should call 911 or give you a glucagon injection, a prescription medication that you inject to raise blood glucose quickly (ask your doctor for a prescription and educate yourself and those around you on how to administer a glucagon injection). Ask your diabetes educator and your doctor what you need to do before this emergency situation happens to you. Explain what help you would need to anyone who might be with you when you have low blood sugar.

It is best to wear or carry medical identification explaining that you have diabetes. If you should pass out when you are away from home, it will get you the help you need more quickly if people know what condition you have.

Carb Counting Makes the Day Go Easier

Counting the carbohydrate in your food is one of the best ways to control your blood sugar. Carbohydrate has the biggest impact on your blood glucose. So if you can predict what this impact will be, you'll have an advantage in matching exercise or medications to your glucose levels. However, carb counting can seem complicated at times and I'll admit that it can get a little tricky. Do whatever you can to talk with a registered dietitian (RD). A good RD can make all of this seem plain as day.

Like I said, carb makes blood sugar rise. Fat and fiber slow down the rise, so it may be high later than you expect. Slowing down the rise also means that you are not hungry so soon after eating.

As you learned in Chapter 2, carbohydrate is in bread, rice, noodles, popcorn, potatoes, fruits, milk, vegetables, and desserts. Yes, I mean the very desserts you know so well.

Sugar is just another carbohydrate. That is why a brownie has about the same effect on your blood sugar that a baked potato does. There are no forbidden foods, and dessert can be part of your meal plan. A lifetime is a long time to go without dessert. The intent of a good treatment plan is not to deny you the enjoyment of eating. Intensive management of diabetes with good control need not become a "thou shall not" experience. You still have to be responsible enough to make wise food choices. To be healthiest, you need to choose more vegetables than dessert, more fresh foods than processed ones. Whole grains and vegetables give you the vitamins, minerals, and fiber you need. They're premium fuel for your body.

It is important for each of us to learn how much carbohydrate is in the food you eat. This way you can try to eat about the same amount of carb at each meal. If two types of food have the same amount of carb, you can switch one for the other without making your blood sugar go too high. For example a piece of bread has about 15 grams of carb. A small apple has about 15 grams of carb. A 1/3 cup serving of rice has about 15 grams of carb. An 8-oz glass of milk has about 15 grams of carb. All of these can be interchanged with one another to give you the same amount of carbohydrate.

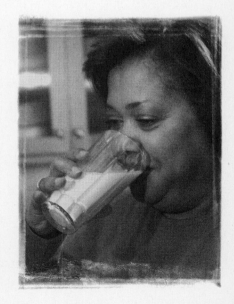

If you are eating a food with a food label—and most fresh fruits and vegetables don't have one—it helps to learn where to look for information about carb and other things, such as the size of the serving and how much saturated fat is in it. To find the carb in foods that don't have labels, buy or check out books from the library that list

Important Fact
Vegetables have only 5 grams of carb in a serving, which is another reason to eat more veggies.

carb and fat gram counts. Some cookbooks, like the ones from the American Diabetes Association, have this information with each recipe, too.

Look at the label in Figure 8-1. You will see that fiber and sugar are part of the Total Carbohydrate on the label. Ignore the grams of sugar, because they're part of the Total Carb. If the food has more than five grams of fiber, you can subtract that number from the Total Carb. This is another benefit of high-fiber foods such as whole grains, fruits, and vegetables. Fiber slows down the rise in blood sugar.

Be sure to double-check the serving size. Many times a box or can of food has two or three servings in it, not just one. The information on the label, however, is for just one serving. If you eat the whole can of food, then you are getting two times as many of the nutrients on the label. Learn what a certain serving size actually looks like by using true measuring devices. For example, my father's idea of a "cup" was the mug from which he drank his coffee. Turns out this was actually 2 1/2 cups! Imagine what the effects of a portion size error like that could be on one's diet (and weight) over time. What is your idea of a cup?

Tricks of the Trade

- Eat nutritious foods. Using a menu or meal plan is a big help. If you prefer, choose your own foods and count calories or carbs.

- Learn how much carbohydrate is in foods, so you don't eat too much at one meal.

Figure 8-1. Reading Food Labels

Nutrition Facts

Serving Size 1 cup (228g)
Servings Per Container 2

Amount Per Serving

Calories 260   Calories from Fat 120

	% Daily Value*
Total Fat 13g	**20%**
Saturated Fat 5g	**25%**
Cholesterol 30mg	**10%**
Sodium 660mg	**28%**
Total Carbohydrate 31g	**10%**
Dietary Fiber 0g	**0%**
Sugars 5g	
Protein 5g	

Vitamin A 4%   •   Vitamin C 2%

Calcium 15%   •   Iron 4%

* Percent Daily Values are based on a 2,000 calorie diet. Your daily values may be higher or lower depending on your calorie needs:

	Calories:	2,000	2,500
Total Fat	Less than	65g	80g
Sat Fat	Less than	20g	25g
Cholesterol	Less than	300mg	300mg
Sodium	Less than	2,400mg	2,400mg
Total Carbohydrate		300g	375g
Dietary Fiber		25g	30g

Calories per gram:
Fat 9 • Carbohydrate 4 • Protein 4

- Exercise daily. Have fun, mix it up, and keep moving to the music.

- Take your medications as your doctor tells you to.

- Check your blood sugar often and record the information you need to make good decisions on behalf of your pancreas, heart, kidneys, eyes, and feet.

Emotions: How We Face It

Everyone with diabetes wants a cure. Every family with diabetes in it wants a cure. It is a disease that gives no breaks, no time outs, no vacations. High blood sugar can make you feel wiped out and unable to cope. High blood sugar can change your personality if you don't watch out. Be kind to yourself and don't expect to be perfect. We are human and the only

The Four Things Others Should Know (Grandparents, Teachers, Bus Drivers)

- If you take insulin or medication that puts you at risk for low blood sugar, know the symptoms of low blood sugar and what to do to treat it. Don't let anyone eat the foods or drinks that are set aside for low-blood sugars. You need them when you need them. Always have them with you, either in the car, at school, at home, on vacation, on trips, everywhere you go, have them handy.
- Know the symptoms of high blood sugar and what to do about it.
- Encourage, praise, and support the person with diabetes. No nagging allowed.
- Choose a healthy lifestyle for yourself, too. It's as good as walking a mile in the other person's shoes.

constant in our lives is that things keep changing. Use blood sugar numbers as a sign to take action. Learn what those actions are. Be understanding of your challenges, and realize how much you are doing!

Burnout

People get burned out if they think they have to do everything the health care provider says and to do it every day. This is not reasonable. You have the freedom to choose what to do—but you need to know what all your choices are. For example, you want to have a piece of birthday cake, but it isn't on your meal plan. Then you can choose either to adjust your insulin or to take a walk. If you don't take insulin, you can eat the cake and skip the bread or rice in your next meal. You can trade one carb for another. You can make adjustments when you know what choices you have available. This type of flexible strategy will keep you in control of the disease.

A dietitian told me of a married couple who came to see her about a month after the husband had been diagnosed with diabetes. The family doctor had torn out a meal plan from a magazine and given it to the man to use until he could get in to see the dietitian. Well, it had cottage cheese for breakfast and all sorts of foods that this little old couple from Georgia were not used to eating. The wife was upset about having to shop for foods that she had never bought before, and the husband had lost 15 pounds but was swearing that he'd rather die than stay on that diet.

A couple of things were going on in this situation. The doctor didn't have time to create a meal plan with foods that the man usually ate—which is what a registered dietitian will do for you. And the couple didn't go to the library or get on the Internet or do anything to try to find other information about the foods he could eat. See Chapter 2. Real Food. A healthy meal is a healthy meal for everyone.

Caregivers: Family, Friends, and Co-Workers of People with Diabetes

People with diabetes have demands on their time and attention beyond what the rest of us have. They can get tired, burned out, stressed, confused, and angry. You want to help, but what can you do? Let them express emotions as they bubble up. Ask, "What is the hardest part for you? What seems to work well?" This reminds them of their strengths. Encourage them to go to support groups, and to talk with the doctor if they are too sad or depressed for long periods of time. Everybody needs help at one time or another.

Diabetes has an effect on your emotions, too. Be honest with how you feel. As your family member or friend changes, you will have to change, too. Being honest can help you both.

You might ask: What do I do that helps with your diabetes? What do I do that makes it harder for you to manage your diabetes? Don't play the "diabetes police," where you constantly hound your loved one and enforce rules and routines. This is an easy role for many people to fall into. Try playing the trusted colleague assisting with problem-solving ideas. For example, offer to go to the doctor with your father or mother. Take a walk with your wife or your child. Cook a special meal that is tasty and healthy for the whole family. These are truly helpful acts.

If you learn more about diabetes, you will understand better what it takes to manage it. There is a lot of guesswork to balancing blood sugar levels. Informed guesses are more helpful.

Make Changes in Small Steps

Change doesn't go in a straight line. Change comes about in small steps up. If you try to take 5 flights of stairs at once, you're likely to fall, and you are not likely to keep doing it even if you make it. Taking the stairs one at a time makes sense. Figure out the steps that you need to take. Ask your doctor or nurse or dietitian for help. If you are not going to do what they suggest—or you don't believe it will work—say so. You live with this plan, so talk it over to figure out what might work for you. This is new ground for you, so you may have to try some new approaches to the way you do things.

Toolkits for Success

Regular maintenance checks are a good idea. Keep a running tab on how the different systems in your body are doing. You want your doctor to catch any problems early, when they can be treated. For example, diabetic eye disease (retinopathy) can be treated with laser surgery, and blindness can be prevented if the problem is found early enough to be treated.

Checkups keep you on the path to good health. You and your health care providers need this information, so you can work together to keep you healthy.

Regular Checkups

The Test	When	Goal	Your Numbers
A1C	Twice a year	Below 7	_____
Blood pressure	At each doctor visit	130/80	_____
LDL cholesterol	Once a year	below 100	_____
Eyes	Yearly dilated eye exam		
Kidneys	Yearly urine test		
Nerves	Yearly check with plastic wire		
Feet	Regularly check for changes in shape and feeling		

Once a Year

- Foot exam. Check for loss of feeling with a plastic wire.

- Dilated eye exam.

- Blood test for creatinine and cholesterol levels.

- Urine check for protein.

- Dental exam.

Diabetes Management Checklist

☐ Exercise. It makes your cells more sensitive to insulin and lowers blood glucose.

☐ Eat right.

☐ If you need to, lose a little weight, say 10 to 15 pounds. Less body means more insulin to go around. People with type 1 diabetes are usually younger and slim. Their bodies don't make any insulin, so this step does not apply to them.

☐ Check your blood sugar regularly. Write the numbers down, see what patterns appear. Is it often high after lunch? Usually low in the morning?

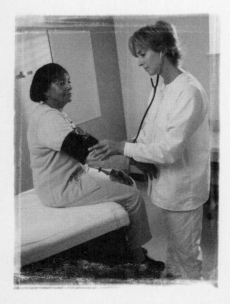

☐ Take all your medications as prescribed.

☐ Talk over your blood glucose records with your doctor or educator to see what is going on. You may need to change your medication or the dose you take. You may need to eat more fiber and fat at breakfast. You may need a different timing for your exercise. Balancing your blood sugar levels is an art, and you are the artist.

Resources

Online

If you are eligible for Medicare, ask your health care provider about diabetes education classes and an appointment with a dietitian. Medicare should help pay for these and for diabetes supplies.
www.medicare.gov

If you have problems paying for food, medicines, and medical supplies, ask your doctor, nurse, or pharmacist to help you find resources. To check on drug assistance programs go to:
www.benefitscheckup.org

Associations

American Diabetes Association
1701 N. Beauregard Street
Alexandria, VA 22311
1-800-DIABETES (342-2383)
www.diabetes.org

Black & Brown Sugar
310 E. Florence Ave
Inglewood, CA 90301
(800) 788-0941
www.blackandbrownsugar.com
Diabetes information for African American, Latino, and other populations at risk for diabetes. Hosted by Lenore T. Coleman, Pharm.D, CDE.

National Diabetes Education Program (NDEP)
1 Diabetes Way
Bethesda, MD 20892-3600
1-800-438-5383
www.ndep.nih.gov

The NDEP offers the free "Foot Care Kit" and "Power to Control Diabetes Kit."

National Institute of Diabetes and Digestive and Kidney Diseases
National Diabetes Information Clearinghouse
1 Information Way
Bethesda, MD 20892-3560
1-800-860-8747
www.niddk.nih.gov/health/diabetes/ndic.htm

Centers for Disease Control and Prevention
Division of Diabetes Translation
1-877-232-3422
www.cdc.gov/diabetes

American Association of Diabetes Educators (AADE)
100 W. Monroe Street, Suite 400
Chicago, Illinois 60603
1-800-Team-UP-4
www.aadenet.org

American Dietetic Association
120 South Riverside Plaza, Suite 2000
Chicago, IL 60606-6995
1-800-366-1655
www.eatright.org

Books and Magazines

Diabetes Burnout, by William H. Polonsky, PhD. American Diabetes Association, 1999. Also available on audiotape.

Getting a Grip on Diabetes: Tips and Techniques for Kids and Teens, by Spike and Bo Loy. American Diabetes Association, 2000.

Diabetes Meal Planning Made Easy, 2nd edition, by Hope Warshaw, MMSc, RD, CDE. American Diabetes Association, 2000.

Diabetes A to Z, 5th edition, by ADA. American Diabetes Association, 2003.

Diabetes Forecast. Monthly magazine published by the American Diabetes Association.

9

KIDNEY DISEASE

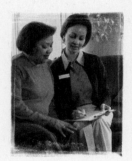

As I mentioned before, we African Americans are more likely to have high blood pressure. We've seen this can have some pretty nasty effects on our hearts, leading to heart attack and stroke. But your heart is not the only vital organ negatively affected by hypertension. It damages your kidneys, too. In fact, African Americans are four times more likely to have kidney disease and, ultimately, kidney failure. This is a serious deadly disease, and we get it way too often. If you have a relative with kidney disease on top of high blood pressure, you're running an incredibly high risk.

Part of the reason kidney disease is so prevalent is because it often doesn't show any symptoms, which means you can have it and not feel it. You need to get a simple urine test every year to find out how your kidneys are doing. Ask for the test. It doesn't hurt at all. It costs about $25 and it can save your life. Many doctors don't automatically request this test, so ask for it. The most accurate results seem to come from the first morning specimen. The National Institutes of Health (NIH) has a pilot program going right now to educate people at risk to save their kidneys. This means you.

The Need to Prevent

High blood pressure damages kidneys so they can't filter wastes from your bloodstream. Many people don't realize it, but you can still urinate just fine, even when your kidneys are failing. That may be the reason why many of the 20 million people with kidney failure don't realize that they have it.

We need to prevent kidney disease because there are few treatments for it once it develops. The frightening fact is that end-stage kidney disease has doubled in the U.S. in the last 10 years, and 400,000 people have it now. This number of sick folks is expected to double again in the next 10 years. Let's stop this trend now.

What Do the Kidneys Do?

The kidneys are two little organs about the size of Idaho potatoes located in the small of the back above your waist on each side of the spine. One can do the work for two, which is why people can give up a kidney for transplants. Their most important job is to filter wastes out of the blood, to maintain the balance of water in the tissues, and to maintain normal blood chemistry. They also manufacture hormones that stimulate the bone marrow to make red blood cells and regulate the absorption of calcium from the intestines. Blood flows through the kidney at a rate of about one quart every minute. The "cleaned" blood moves on and the wastes leave your body as urine.

Some people who are at risk don't have protein in their urine or retinopathy (eye disease) either, both of which are the signs that point to kidney damage. But they do have kidney damage. The only way to discover this damage is with a simple blood test checking the glomerular filtration rate (GFR), which shows whether the kidneys are filtering as they should. If you have high blood pressure or diabetes or a family member with kidney disease, you should ask your doctor for this test. There is more information about this at the National Kidney and Urologic Diseases Information Clearinghouse site (see Resources at the end of the chapter for contact information).

Preventing Kidney Disease

If you reach end-stage kidney failure you need dialysis or a kidney transplant to stay alive. So, what can you do to prevent this from happening?

- Lower your cholesterol.

- Lower your blood pressure.

- If applicable, control your diabetes.

You make your best start on doing all three with a daily 30-minute walk and eating better. There are also good medications to help you with all three conditions.

Men and Their Cholesterol Levels

So, you're thinking to yourself, "I'm a healthy male, I don't have diabetes or high blood pressure, so I'm okay." What about your cholesterol levels?

If you have high LDL (bad) cholesterol and low HDL (good) cholesterol, you're twice as likely to have kidney disease. Lifestyle affects these levels, too. And there are some medications that can help you as well. Do what you need to do to keep yourself healthy.

Remember that it doesn't hurt until it's too late to do much about it. Don't wait for symptoms to show up. Know your risk and have it checked out. End-stage kidney failure is preventable if you know early on that your kidneys are having problems.

Protein in Your Urine?

If you have had the urine test and you do have protein in your urine, you can start taking a blood pressure drug that can slow down the damage to your kidneys. The first choice would be either angiotensin II receptor blockers (ARBs) or angiotensin converting enzyme (ACE) inhibitors. Both of these pills relax tiny blood vessels in the kidneys. Talk with your doctor about which one would work best for you. A small number of people develop a dry cough as a side effect and have to stop taking the drug, but it may well be that most people with diabetes need to be taking one of these drugs.

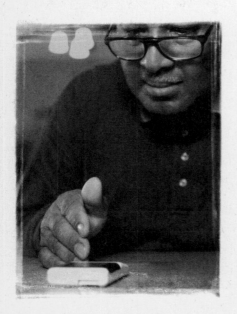

If you have diabetes, getting it under control is crucial, too. Diabetes is the leading cause of kidney failure, but if you maintain good blood glucose control you can beat the odds. Of people with type 1 diabetes, about a third are at risk for kidney disease (nephropathy) after having had diabetes for more than 40 years. With type 2 diabetes, kidney failure is a bit of a mystery and seems to be a sign that the person is at risk for a stroke or heart attack.

Dipstick-Positive Proteinuria

At the next stage in the disease, you are losing so much protein in your urine that you don't have enough albumin (protein) in your bloodstream to hold plasma water inside the blood vessels. This causes you to get swollen feet and ankles and hands at this stage. The water accumulates in the tissues, causing swelling or edema. It can collect around the heart and in the abdomen, too. This is when you may start to get some symptoms of the disease. Water weight may reach 50 pounds. This weight makes you tired and short of breath. People with this syndrome often notice that their shoes don't fit and dresses and pants will not button because of the water weight.

Chronic Kidney Failure

This is the end-stage of the disease, as the kidneys can no longer filter all the toxins from the blood. Your doctor may continue to monitor urine and blood tests to see what chemicals are getting through. If your serum creatinine level rises above two, you should see a kidney specialist. This level of the disease is usually marked by the appearance of noticeable symptoms, such as:

- Listlessness

- Loss of appetite

- Feeling cold

- Mental confusion

- Nausea

- Itching

- Anemia

After some years, the person with kidney failure will need either dialysis or a kidney transplant to live.

What Is Dialysis?

Dialysis uses a machine (an artificial kidney) to clean the waste products from your blood. There must be a connection put in place in a blood vessel, usually in your arm, so your blood can flow to the machine. This method of dialysis, called hemodialysis, is usually done three times a week and takes four to six hours each time.

Another form of dialysis, called peritoneal dialysis, removes wastes from the blood in the small blood vessels in the membrane lining your abdominal cavity. After the doctor creates a permanent connection here, a cleaning solution can be put into and drained out of the abdomen at regular intervals. About two liters of solution are put into the abdomen and drained out every four to six hours. Although not many people use this type of dialysis, if you are highly motivated and trained to do it, you don't have to keep going in to the clinic three times a week.

A kidney transplant can heal you. However, it is an expensive operation and will not be an option for older people who are very ill with other diseases. Further, once you have a transplanted organ, you must take powerful drugs to suppress the action of your immune system, which will try to kill the foreign tissue in your body.

What Else Can Harm Your Kidneys?

Some over the counter medications, such as ibuprofen (Advil, Motrin, and others) and naproxen (Aleve), can harm your kidneys. Prescription antibiotics such as cisplatin and psychiatric medications such as lithium can also cause damage. There are many prescription anti-inflammatory drugs that can damage your kidneys, too. Ask your physician and pharmacist if a drug will harm your kidneys.

If you have an x-ray done, the dye used can cause kidney damage. If you must have a dye study done, for example before heart bypass surgery, you can be given IV fluids and certain drugs before and after the procedure to help your kidneys withstand the stress.

If your bladder does not empty normally, it can make urine back up into your kidneys and damage them. The only sign may be a fever or a backache. Pay attention and get the condition treated as soon as possible.

Meal Plans Are Important

You'll need to work with a dietitian on a meal plan. You need a diet lower in fats, cholesterol, and protein. You may also need to eat less salt (sodium), potassium, or phosphorus. We actually only need about one half teaspoon of salt a day to maintain the fluid balance in our bodies. Edema (swelling of the feet and legs) happens when your kidneys cannot filter and remove the salt. It is a sign of kidney damage. If your kidneys are struggling, you may need to eat less protein to ease the demand you are putting on them. The current recommendation is 40 to 60 grams of protein a day. If you cut back to that amount, it has an almost immediate beneficial effect on your kidneys.

The National Kidney Foundation has many informative pamphlets, but one, *Dining Out with Confidence*, can help you make healthy food choices at home and when eating out. One of the problems with soul food is that it can be high in sodium, phosphorus, potassium, and fat. Take care not to eat too much salted and cured meat such as bacon or sausages. Your best choices, says the pamphlet, may be "fried chicken (with skin removed), corn, string beans or okra, wilted lettuce, corn bread, butter, and sweet potato pie (small wedge)."

The Bottom Line
Don't give up.

Resources

Online

Learn more about the National Kidney Disease Education Program at:
www.nkdep.nih.gov/getkid.htm

Associations

National Kidney Foundation
30 East 33rd Street
New York, NY 10016
800-622-9010
www.kidney.org

National Kidney and Urologic Diseases Information Clearinghouse
3 Information Way
Bethesda, MD 20892-3580
800-891-5390
www.niddk.nih.gov/health/kidney/kidney.htm

Division of Organ Transplantation
Office of Special Programs
Health Resources and Services Administration
Parklawn Building, Room 7C-22
5600 Fishers Lane
Rockville, MD 20857
301-443-7577
www.organdonor.gov

10

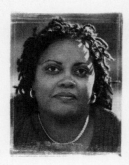

CANCER AND WHAT YOU CAN DO ABOUT IT

Cancer happens when cells in the body stop behaving normally and grow out of control, forming a tumor. Your body's immune system is always on the lookout for these abnormal changes in cells, and it's possible your body may be defeating cancer cells more often than we know. However, your immune system can get overwhelmed. That is the best reason to learn how you can strengthen and support your body's natural disease fighting system (see the Chapter 2. Real Food and Chapter 3. Being Active Is Being Alive).

The Power of Prevention

A lot about cancer is still unknown, but there is evidence that environmental factors, such toxins in the air, radiation, and others, can act as a trigger to get the cancer ball rolling. This is why a strong natural defense system is the key to cancer prevention. Your immune

> Stop smoking. It's not cool. It kills you. Period.

system can become overwhelmed by the toxins and stress around you and in you. Then the immune system cannot destroy the cancer cells when they begin to grow. The key to cancer is prevention. Help your immune system help you. Good food (lots of vegetables and whole grains), daily exercise, and losing weight if you need to, help prevent cancer of all kinds.

Check Your Environment

Ask yourself the following questions:

- Do you live near any places where substances that are known to cause cancer can build up, such as a dump or high-tension wires?

- Do you live with a lot of stress? Are you very ill, very poor, or living with people who are angry or violent? All of these cause stress. Stress hormones are powerful, and you want to turn them off when you can.

- Do you have high blood pressure?

- Do you smoke?

- Do you take drugs or drink too much alcohol?

- Do you have impaired glucose tolerance (IGT)? People with higher than normal insulin levels in their blood because of IGT are more likely to develop cancer. They are twice as likely to die of any cancer, 4 times as likely to have colon cancer, 50% as likely to die of lung cancer. But the research shows that people with outright diabetes did not have these risks. Losing weight and exercising help your body use insulin better and lower the risk.

Preventing Cancer in the Young

Young women who eat lots of red meat and whole milk increase their chances of breast cancer. Do American children and teenagers eat much else? Research shows that three to four hours of moderate exercise a week can cut a woman's risk of breast cancer by 40%. It's most protective if you start this daily walking when you are a teenager. These are things you can do to protect your daughters.

Preventing Cancer in Ourselves

Obesity increases your chances of getting breast, colon, and uterine cancers. It also inclines you toward cervical, ovarian, pancreatic, and liver cancer. Bulging waistlines in women contribute to 20% of all cancer deaths. The connection is thought to be in fat cells, which may produce hormone-like substances that encourage tumor growth. Men with a bulging

---

Cancer Prevention Toolkit

- Lose weight.
- Eat fruits and vegetables, beans, and whole grains. The antioxidants and fiber protect you.
- Take a walk every day.
- Share your feelings with a friend or family member.
- Check your environment for cancer-causing chemicals, etc.
- Learn relaxation techniques to deal with stress and encourage your immune system.

belly are at risk for colon, prostate, pancreatic, and liver cancer. Let's lose some weight for the cancer prevention it gives.

Treating Cancer

If you get cancer, find as much information about the disease as you can. There are support groups and associations with the information you need to make decisions about what treatments you believe will work for you. If you don't believe it will work, don't try it.

Cancer research is intense and well funded, so much is being learned every day. However, there are currently only three common methods to try to treat cancer:

- Surgery

- Radiation

- Chemotherapy

If the cancer is all in one place, surgery can cut it out. This works pretty well. Radiation and chemotherapy are supposed to kick the immune system into high gear, to defeat the cancer. Unfortunately, radiation and chemotherapy are so strong that they kill many normal cells and do a lot of damage to the body. They may not get the immune system going again. As of right now there are no sure cures for cancer.

Some people find that changing to a different diet, such as a high-fiber vegetarian diet, and staying away from sugar, alcohol, tobacco, and red meat helps their immune system get going again. That is the key, to encourage the immune system to get back in the game because it is your body's perfect healing tool.

Getting regular exercise, especially walking outside and breathing deeply in fresh air, will make you feel better and get your circulation and digestion moving more normally. Everything that you do to be healthier is noticed immediately by your body and appreciated.

The Healing Power of Pictures

We've all seen movies and television shows. These are moving pictures, images that the actors and director guide us to see. It's good that we've had some practice, because research shows that the images we create in our mind and feel in our body can help us heal. It sounds a little strange and hard to believe, but it's true. Call it biofeedback or guided imagery, it is a tool that may be helpful for you.

Biofeedback helps you listen to your body through machines that indicate with a light or sound when certain physical changes, such as dropping blood pressure or slowing heart rate, occurs within your body. With practice you can learn to feel the subtle changes that lead to a drop in blood pressure, so you can make them happen. If you have high blood pressure, you may imagine your blood vessels as relaxed and elastic and the blood flowing smoothly through them. You might put your hand on your heart and see it beating slowly. The machine tells you if you are, in fact, lowering your blood pressure. With practice, you can do it when you need to without having to have feedback from the machine. Biofeedback can help relieve pain, too. The pictures you hold in your mind work with your body in this.

The most extensive research of this technique has been done on the effect of guided imagery on cells. People have been successful in boosting their immune system, which can be measured in blood and saliva. In a study by Mark Rider, Ph.D., and Jeanne Achterberg, Ph.D., patients used guided imagery to tell the immune system to attack certain cells and to leave others alone. With a little understanding of cellular activity this can be very effective. It isn't hard to learn how cells work, and it can help you more clearly visualize the action and the positive effect that you want.

Guided imagery has assisted people in preparing for surgery, with the outcome that they healed quickly and with less pain than expected. The effectiveness of guided imagery with cancer patients has been shown in several well-designed studies. In one such study conducted at UCLA, patients with malignant melanoma participated in a six-week class teaching stress management, communication, and mind/body skills (guided imagery). This group had 1/4 the number of deaths and less than 1/2 as many recurrences of the cancer in the next five years.

If you want to learn more about guided imagery and what you might do with it, check the resources at the end of this chapter, go online, or head to the library. Hesitancy is understandable with something like this, but don't let fear of the unknown keep you from helping yourself or the ones you love. Guided imagery can't hurt you, and it just might help.

Your Faith

A life-threatening disease, like cancer, usually brings folks face to face with their faith or their lack of it. Faith has moved mountains and healed cancer, too. Even if you don't believe, this may be the time to ask the local church prayer group to pray for you. Research shows that prayer on behalf of others has an effect, even if they don't know they are being prayed for.

Resources

General

Many universities and hospitals have their own cancer research centers. If you live near a university or hospital, this may be a good place to start looking for information.

Educate yourself. Visit a medical library and look up the treatments for your condition. Get online and explore the many resources available to you.

Online

For a thoughtfully planned and nourishing place that offers information about therapies, resources, and emotional support to people with cancer and their families, visit: *www.touchedbycancer.org*

Another comprehensive website for cancer can be found at: *www.canceronline.com*

Prostate cancer is higher in African American men. For more information go to: *www.cdc.gov/cancer/prostate/prostate.htm*

You can order free materials at: *http://webapp.cdc.gov/IXPRESS/PUBSPROD/DCPC+ BOOK/DCPC1.DML*

A selection of guided imagery audio tapes are available from the Academy of Guided Imagery: *www.interactiveimagery. com*

Associations

American Cancer Society
1599 Clifton Road, NE
Atlanta, GA 30329
800-227-2345
www.cancer.org

Cancer Information Service
National Cancer Institute
9000 Rockville Pike
Bethesda, MD 20892
800-4-CANCER (800-422-6237)
http://cis.nci.nih.gov
www.cancer.gov

Cancer Research Foundation of America
1600 Duke Street, Suite 110
Alexandria, VA 22314
800-227-2732
www.preventcancer.org

African American Breast Cancer Alliance
P.O. Box 8981
Minneapolis, MN 55408
www.geocities.com/aabcainc

Susan G. Komen Breast Cancer Foundation
5005 LBJ Freeway
Dallas, TX 75244
800-462-9273
www.komen.org

The Academy of Guided Imagery
P.O. Box 2070
Mill Valley, CA 94942
800-726-2070
www.interactiveimagery.com

Books

Guided Imagery Resources:

Staying Well with Guided Imagery: How to Harness the Power of Your Imagination for Health and Healing, by Belleruth Naparstek. Warner Books, 1995.

Guided Imagery for Self-Healing, by Martin L. Rossman, MD. H.J. Kramer, 2000.

The various works of Dean Ornish, MD, Larry Dossey, MD, and Joan Borysenko, PhD.

11

WOMEN'S ISSUES

Women are susceptible to a variety of health issues that men will never have to consider. Men may be more prone to high blood pressure, heart attack and the like, but they'll also never have to worry about having an ovarian cyst. There's a reason an entire branch of medicine is devoted solely to women's health issues. You have an organic system tucked into your body—a system designed to produce life—which men do not. Of course, this isn't the only thing that sets you apart from men in terms of health. There are a variety of issues unrelated to childbearing that are specific to women. In this chapter, I'll cover a few.

The Importance of a Healthy Pregnancy

Mothers are the most important people in the health of the entire family, but especially of the children. What you eat and your level of

fitness are as important to your children's health as it is to
your own. This is both the honor and the long-reaching
responsibility that you were given at birth.

Mothers who don't eat well before pregnancy don't have
the stores of calcium and other nutrients that they and their
babies need. That's why the old wives' tale says that you lose
a tooth for every baby. For many nutrients your body gives
the baby whatever it has, and you get whatever is left. You
and your developing baby deserve the best food. Again vegetables, fruit, lean meat, and whole grains are the way to go.
Drink lots of water and take a daily walk. Taking time to be
outside to feel the sun on your face and enjoy the slower
rhythms of nature can soothe you. Learn to breathe deeply
and slowly to energize and relax your body. You know it
works during labor, but I'm telling you that your breathing
has great power all the time.

Mothers who don't eat well during pregnancy might have
babies who don't weigh enough, and who haven't had a
chance to develop their organs as well as they should have.
Both low birth weight and high birth weight can lead to diabetes in the baby. If a mother has diabetes while she is pregnant and her blood sugar levels are high throughout the
pregnancy, her child grows in a high-sugar environment and
is more likely to get diabetes. If that baby is a girl, she is then
more likely to grow up to have a child with diabetes, too. You
see the powerful effect your choices have on the generations
of children and grandchildren who arrive here through you.

If you have diabetes, take care not to get pregnant until
you are ready, until your blood sugar is under control. This
will keep you and your baby as safe and as healthy as possible. It can prevent birth defects. And prevention is what we
are all about.

As soon as you find out that you are pregnant, see a health
care provider. Most pregnancies go smoothly, but to protect
your health and the health of the baby, get there early and

stay in touch with your provider all the way through. It is wise not to smoke or to drink alcohol while you are pregnant. It is wise not to take any drugs, but if you are on a prescription that is important for your own health, such as blood pressure medication, discuss what to do with your doctor. You may need to change the type and dose of your medication to keep your baby healthy. Women who have type 2 diabetes will need to take insulin injections during the pregnancy if diet is not enough to keep blood glucose levels under control. Diabetes pills are not approved for pregnant women—we don't know how they might affect the baby.

A nurse educator or dietitian can help you learn to balance food, exercise, and insulin, so your blood sugar stays balanced. The dietitian can help you design a meal plan and to make changes to the meal plan as the pregnancy progresses. Breastfeeding goes better if you know what to eat and how much. And, of course, a meal plan can help you lose weight after the baby is weaned. You'll find that your body holds onto about 10 extra pounds while you are breastfeeding. That's its way of insuring there's enough for the baby in case of famine or you get sick. The body's wisdom was developed over thousands of years, and we are not going to convince it to let go of those last 10 pounds until it is ready. When the baby is weaned, you don't need it anymore.

After Birth—Breastfeeding

Breastfeeding is nature's way of providing for the child's best nutrition. It's not just more convenient and easier for you than handling all those bottles. Breastfeeding gives your baby a head start on good health by providing him with your grown-up immunities to disease.

Breastfeeding your baby for 6–12 months reduces the child's risk of being obese and of getting type 2 diabetes. You are the only one who can give this magical gift. If this isn't motivation enough for you, breastfeeding also makes a calmer, happier child who is less likely to get into trouble with the law in later years. We even have research on that!

If you choose to feed your baby formula, please check the ingredients label to be sure that it contains omega-3 fatty acids. These fats are vital to your child's brain function and help with better vision, too.

Good Fats and Fish and Mercury

When you are pregnant or breastfeeding, you should not eat certain fish because the levels of mercury in some fish can be damaging to your baby (see Chapter 2. Real Food). Mercury damages the brain and nerves. Adults can stop eating tuna or whichever fish is mercury-laden, and in a few weeks or so, the body will clear the mercury with no lasting ill effects. However, small children and babies still growing in their mothers can suffer permanent brain damage from mercury. Don't expose them to it if you can help it.

A Word about the News, Magazines, and Health Shows on TV

Make sure you get your health information from good sources. You may not be getting the information you need from the media or from public service advertisements. Breast cancer and AIDS get lots of attention, but heart disease is the number one killer of women, not breast cancer. Only 4% of women die of breast cancer, but 45% die of cardiovascular disease. In fact, you are more likely to have heart disease, a sexually transmitted disease, or depression than you are to have breast cancer. I'm not saying breast cancer isn't serious. But know what diseases you are truly at risk for and then do something to prevent them or at least slow them down!

Birth Control

It would be best for your health and the baby's if you don't get pregnant until you want to. And yet, we know that the best birth control methods are still only 99% effective. Do your best. Preventing a pregnancy 99 times out of 100 is still a heck of a lot better than doing nothing at all.

You have several choices in birth control, and you need to discuss which one is for you with your doctor and your partner. Obviously, if you are not married and you have several sexual partners, you want to choose a birth control method that will protect you against sexually transmitted diseases (STDs) too.

There are basically two types of birth control—the barrier methods that prevent the sperm from getting to the egg, and the hormone methods that trick the body into thinking that it is already pregnant, so it won't allow another one to take place.

- **The Pill**—This is the best known hormone method. It is effective for many women, but in research studies, 1 to 8 women in every 100 still get pregnant on the pill. The pill also does not protect you against STDs. It may aggravate high blood pressure or your chances of a stroke. The hormones in the pill may help protect you against some female cancers, but they may also cause you to have bloating, nausea, or other symptoms of PMS or pregnancy. Those hormones are powerful and each woman will react to them in her own way.

- **The Condom**—A condom is a barrier method, perhaps the most popular one in the world. It prevents the sperm from traveling up the vagina to the egg, and it prevents STDs. There are larger condoms made for women that may provide better protection against STDs because they cover more of the opening to the vagina. Condoms are made of latex and polyurethane. Polyurethane may work better for people who are allergic to latex.

- **The Diaphragm**—This is another barrier method, as it blocks the path that the sperm takes to get to the egg. You put a jelly inside the diaphragm that kills sperm, which increases the effectiveness of this method. Maybe twice as many women get pregnant with a diaphragm as the number who take pills (16 out of 100), but you do not have the side effects. After you have had a baby, you may need to be fitted for a different sized diaphragm. It can press on your urethra, so to prevent a bladder infection urinate before and after you have sex. It does not protect against STDs.

- **The Sponge**—This is not as effective as the other barrier methods, and it does not protect you against STDs. It is convenient and inexpensive. If you use it with a condom, your chances of not conceiving are better.

- **The Ring**—This is a new device. It is a ring that releases hormones when you put it around your cervix. You leave it on for three weeks and then take it out for one week to allow a period to happen. You need a prescription for this, as you do with the pill, and you have the same risks that you do with the pill. Use a condom for protection from STDs.

- **The IUD**—An IUD has to be placed in your cervix by a doctor, but then you do nothing else but occasionally check that it is still in place. An IUD is more effective than the pill or the ring, and does not carry their health risks. New IUDs may release some hormones but at such low doses that they do not cause the clotting or stroke risk. IUDs can stay in place for five years, and when you are ready to start trying to have a baby, sim-

ply have it removed. IUDs can cause heavy bleeding
with periods.

- **The Progesterone Shot**—This is a hormone injection
  that you get every three months. It is an effective birth
  control method because you can't forget to take it.
  Again, hormones are powerful and may have side
  effects, such as bloating, headache, weight gain, and
  bleeding. Like the other hormone methods, the shot
  does not protect against STDs.

- **The Patch**—The patch stays on for one week and
  releases hormones into your body. It has the same risks
  and side effects as the pill. You still need a condom for
  STD protection.

- **Emergency Contraception**—If you have unprotected
  sex, say the condom breaks, you can get a set of pills
  from your doctor containing estrogen and progesterone,
  the hormones in birth control pills, but in higher
  amounts. If you take these pills within 3 days of having
  unprotected sex, you are less likely to get pregnant.
  These are called "morning-after" pills. You might ask
  your doctor for a prescription. Then, if you need emergency contraception, you have it.

Sexually Transmitted Diseases

Sexually transmitted diseases are as popular as ever, even
though there are ways to prevent them. Many women have
absolutely no symptoms to tell them that they are infected.
Please be responsible for your own health and the health of
your partner and protect yourself. Some STDs can be passed
on to babies in the birth process, so do this for the children,
too. This advice is as good for teens as it is for a 50-something
newly divorced mother of three. Wearing or using a

condom—every time—is a good first step, but it can't protect you from every disease. There are condoms made especially for females as well as for males. If you're too embarrassed to buy condoms, as many women are, you can buy them at a drugstore online, such as *www.drugstore.com.*

STDs can be caused by bacteria or by viruses. Some of them, like HPV and herpes, can be transmitted even without sexual intercourse. If you engage in oral sex, you can protect yourself with dental dams or condoms. This helps prevent HIV and chlamydia being passed on this way. If you get an STD caused by bacteria, your doctor can write a prescription for antibiotics for you and your partner. If you get one of the viral STDs, ask your doctor what to do to prevent passing it on. The different STDs are described later in this section.

Many women are afraid to ask their partners about his sexual history. Some are afraid to be honest about their own sexual history, especially if it involves rape or abuse. It's the 21st century. Let us all agree that the question will be asked and answered. If you can't be honest, this relationship isn't very important. A self-respecting woman like you deserves an honest answer, too. Find out about his health before you find out any more. Yes, you are worth it. Don't be embarrassed to get the help you need from your doctor. It is your own body; you must speak up on its behalf.

Pap Smears and STD Screening

You should have a check up and Pap smear every two to three years, unless you have abnormal results. To get the best results, schedule your Pap about a week after your period is over. Pap smears help protect you by detecting cervical cancer. They do not detect STDs, however, so if you think you might have one—and any time you have unprotected sex, you might have one—you need to ask your doctor for screening tests. The tests are different for each one, whether it is human papilloma virus (HPV), hepatitis, chlamydia, or HIV/AIDS.

The Centers for Disease Control and Prevention (CDC) recommend that doctors do screenings based on the patient's sexual activity, at pregnancy, or when an STD seems to be going around the neighborhood. But many doctors do not bring up the subject, so you may have to. If you suspect that you have an STD, talk to a doctor. Please don't let feeling embarrassed keep you from getting medication. Most STDs respond well to treatment, so get help as quickly as you can.

If you want to get pregnant, you need STD screening. Several STDs, such as gonorrhea and chlamydia, can scar your fallopian tubes and interfere with you getting pregnant. Active sores of herpes can harm a baby during delivery, too.

The List of STDs

- **Syphilis**—Syphilis is not as common as it once was, but it is still around. There are few symptoms at the beginning, maybe a sore on your genitals or a rash on hands and feet. Over the next six months, you may have muscle pains and hair loss. If it is not treated, it can damage every organ in your body. It is caused by bacteria, so it can be treated with penicillin for you and your partner.

- **Chlamydia**—This may cause pain or discharge or bleeding, but it also may not have any symptoms. You and your partner both need antibiotics to clear this up. Otherwise, he will give it back to you.

- **Gonorrhea**—This may have the same symptoms as chlamydia, which appear about 10 days after exposure. You and your partner both need to take antibiotics.

- **Trichomoniasis**—You may have a vaginal discharge that is greenish-yellow and smells bad. You may have pain on intercourse or urination. You and your partner need the antibiotic metronidazole.

- **Human Papillomavirus (HPV)**—HPV is very common in women and men who are sexually active. This virus can lead to cancer of the cervix, which is discovered when your Pap smear shows abnormal cells. Women over 30 may want to have the DNA Pap smear, which is an HPV test and a Pap. You may develop genital warts or you may not have symptoms. This one is caused by a virus. Ask your doctor what you can do to keep from passing it on, and to control it as much as possible.

- **Hepatitis B**—This is much more common than HIV, but is transmitted the same way. Use condoms, avoid contact involving blood, and get the hepatitis B vaccine. It requires three shots spread out over several months, but all sexually active people should get it. The vaccine is now given to newborn babies. Many people have no symptoms of hepatitis. Some have nausea, vomiting, tiredness, and jaundice. Both hepatitis B and hepatitis C can damage your liver. Your liver is vitally important to balance your blood sugar levels and to filter the toxins out of your body. It can regenerate much of itself, but you need to do all you can to avoid damaging it. You can't live without it.

- **Genital herpes**—This STD is caused by a virus. It shows up as blister-like sores, but it can also make you feel like you have the flu, with body aches and headache. Your doctor can prescribe anti-viral drugs to help control the outbreak. You can pass the virus on to a partner at any time, so always use condoms—male or female condoms—and do not have sex at all when the sores are active. Although they are different viruses,

Other Things That Can Cause Pain, Itching, and Agony

- **Yeast infection**—This infection is caused by an over-growth of yeast, which shows up as white patches on inflamed red skin inside and around the opening to the vagina. Usually, a yeast infection is accompanied by extreme itching and discomfort. Some people buy over the counter medications to treat yeast infections, but if you have done this several times and the condition keeps coming back, you should see a doctor. You may not have a yeast infection, but something else, like a bacterial infection (which is much more common) that needs to be treated with a prescription drug. Yeast infections may show up after you have taken a course of antibiotics for another disease, because the antibiotics also kill the good bacteria that keep the yeast in check. You can try eating yogurt with active bacteria cultures in it to replace the good bacteria that you lost.

- **Hysterectomy**—If your doctor says that you need a hys-terectomy, ask her to list all the alternative treatments. Get a second opinion. This operation was once very common, but may not be necessary for you now. If the reason for the hysterectomy is fibroids, ask about new treatments such as a myomectomy, which removes only the fibroid and leaves young women able to have children after the surgery.

- **Improper technique**—Here's a tip: after you go to the bathroom, be sure to wipe from the front to the back. It prevents bacteria from getting in places you don't want them to go. This helps prevent vaginal infections and cysts.

cold sores can be passed on to your vagina during oral sex, so avoid it until the sores are gone.

- **Genital warts**—These are also caused by a virus. They feel bumpy and may go away on their own. Your doctor may prescribe a cream or remove them with a laser. They are one of the symptoms of HPV. You need a Pap smear.

- **HIV**—Symptoms that you have this virus can take years to show up and when they do, they're in the form of fatigue, weight loss, fever, or headaches. Healthy lifestyle changes and medications are helping people to live longer and longer with this disease. We cannot yet cure HIV and AIDS, but we can sure try to prevent them. Use condoms. Be particular about your sexual partners. Use common sense to keep yourself healthy.

Women and Diabetes

One in every four African American women over 55 has diabetes. Look around; if you have diabetes, you're in good

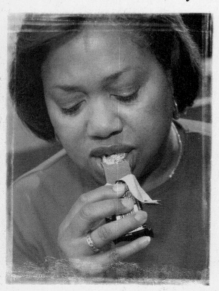

company. Every one of these women need to make the same life changes you do. You may have heard that Oprah is now making those changes, because her mother has diabetes, and Oprah has been diagnosed with pre-diabetes. About half the people diagnosed with pre-diabetes go on to develop full-blown diabetes, but even pre-diabetes can do some nasty stuff if you ignore it.

You and Oprah can lead the way. She may have a chef and a personal trainer, but you're more independent than that. You can make your changes without needing a staff to take care of you. Start low, go slow, and use your common sense.

On the diet that Suzanne Somers created for her, Oprah is eating mainly chicken, fish, vegetables, and fruit. There is nothing wrong with adding a piece of stone-ground cornbread to your dinner, because it tastes good, and it's good for you. Notice, however, that Oprah does not have white flour or sugar in her meals. That is a powerful step toward better health. If you take the white flour and sugar out of your family's meals, what is left on the plate? Check out Chapter 2. Real Food for some suggestions and ideas.

If you will schedule time in your busy day to take a walk—30 minutes to an hour—you will give yourself a new lease on life. This will benefit your health, your attitude, your energy level, your weight, and your family. If you are taking medications for high blood pressure or cholesterol, exercise can help you cut back or get free of them.

Women are more likely than men to be overweight. I'm not sure whether that's because you're taking care of everyone else, or because women think they're too busy to workout, but you can change all that in your life. Your choices count.

How Not to Get Diabetes

Women make up more than half of the 17 million people with diabetes. Your gender, your race, your age, and your family all put you at risk for getting diabetes. Lifestyle changes (eating right and getting to a healthy weight) cuts your risk of diabetes cleanly in half. The Diabetes Prevention Program (DPP) proved that exercise and healthy food choices are the key. Better even than taking a drug called metformin, which is used to treat diabetes. People who lose weight and exercise rule. Changing your attitude about living and eating is the way to conquer diabetes.

Taking Care of Our Girls

Take care of your daughters. Our future lives in them. If your daughter is overweight or obese, she is at risk of serious medical problems, and so are any children she may someday have. If she is entering puberty and she is overweight, she may have polycystic ovarian disease (PCOS). Girls with polycystic ovaries are more likely to develop Metabolic Syndrome (see page 117). It's a very important warning signal. Overweight teen girls are also more likely to develop diabetes. And their babies are more likely to develop diabetes. Good nutrition and daily physical activity can turn off this dire threat to their health and to the health of the next generations. It seems simple, but you have the challenge of getting both yourself and her out and moving.

Physical activity develops more than her muscles; it develops her well-being. It keeps her body happy. An active, healthy girl develops a new sense of who she is and what she can do. Self-confidence comes from physical activity, too.

I recently read of one mother and her 14-year-old daughter who meet regularly in a boxing ring for a work-out that does them good in the ring and at home, too. Get creative with the gifts you have been given and have some fun with your children. They need good nutrition yes, but just as much, they need our attention, our time, our praise, our affection, our respect, and our trust.

One more thing: Black women who get in shape and lower their cholesterol levels well before they reach the age of 55 are giving themselves health insurance of the highest quality. You may never need to take medication to lower cholesterol. It is never too early for you and your daughters to start investing in this program.

Osteoporosis and Supplements to Consider

Women have a challenge to get enough calcium for their bodies. It's an important mineral for the functioning of the body, especially the bones. Bones do more than hold you up, the bone marrow makes red blood cells and the white blood cells that fight off disease for your immune system.

To get the most benefits from calcium, you need more than just calcium itself. You need vitamin D, which you get from sunshine and in supplemented milk, to help you absorb the calcium. You also need magnesium to absorb calcium. However, magnesium is not easy to get from food. Avocados, spinach and other leafy greens, beans, whole grains, and nuts all contain magnesium, but you may need more, especially if you are not eating those foods. You might try a capsule combining calcium and magnesium in a two-to-one ratio, for example: 500 milligrams calcium to 250 milligrams magnesium. Current recommendations are:

- Postmenopausal women should get 1,500 mg of calcium.

- Premenopausal women need 1,000 mg of calcium.

- In all ages, magnesium will help you absorb it better.

Flax seed ground up and sprinkled on cereal, in milkshakes, into baking mixes, and over salads is another food that provides powerful nutrition with a good balance of polyunsaturated fats—omega-3 and omega-6 fatty acids. Sprinkled on food, ground flax seed has a mild, nutty taste. You can also swallow flax seed oil capsules. You don't get the fiber of the seeds, but you do get the healthy fats that work together to lower blood pressure, inflammation, and other vital processes at the level of the cells. Research has shown that flax seeds and the oil have beneficial effects on chronic diseases—all the ones you want to avoid. Talk to your doctor before you start supplementing your diet with flax seed, since it has plant estrogens that may not be healthy for some women.

Hormone Replacement Therapy

You have probably heard about a research study called the Women's Health Initiative (WHI), which seemed to show that the risks of hormone replacement therapy (HRT or HT) outweigh the benefits. This is one of those times when the research is controversial and health care professionals do not agree on the results. No one wants to be a guinea pig, but you have to pay attention to what you think works for you.

There a variety of reasons a woman might take hormone pills are. Some common reasons include:

- Relief of the symptoms of menopause, such as flushes, sleep disturbance, and moodiness

- Osteoporosis

- Vaginal dryness

- Cardiovascular benefits

- Macular degeneration

- Tooth loss

- Skin tone and texture

These may or may not be helped by hormone replacement. The WHI trial was the first one to show that estrogen does prevent fractures and osteoporosis. The cardiovascular benefits—to protect against heart disease and stroke—were not shown. In fact, there may be greater risk of these events with hormone replacement. It's still not clear.

Heart Disease in Women

You've probably seen or read that a woman runs a lower
risk for heart disease, heart attack, and stroke than a man.
This is true. This doesn't mean that it's not a possibility.
Heart disease is still the number one killer of women in this
country. Please protect your heart so you can keep on loving. A woman's symptoms of heart attack are different from
a man's. Look at the symptoms of a heart attack on page
144. Pay close attention to the symptoms that a woman is
most likely to exhibit. You may only feel extremely tired or
sick to your stomach. Pay attention, because the signals
may be subtle. If you are not on a blood thinner like
Coumadin, ask your doctor if you should be taking an
aspirin every day to protect your heart.

If you are taking hormone pills and you want to stop, you
don't have to taper your dose to get off. You're either on or
off. You can quit whenever you want to. If you are consider-
ing HRT, you need to weigh the benefits and risks to you
with your health care team and decide which of the different
HRT combinations might work for you. If you don't want to
try HRT, you might take the advice of JoAnn Manson, MD, a
WHI researcher, who says that 30 minutes a day of physical
activity is much closer to a magic bullet for your health than
popping hormone pills.

What the Doctor Needs to Know

It helps if you know more about your body, how it works,
what it needs, and what illnesses it might get. When you go to
your doctor then, you'll be more in charge of the meeting
between you, and are more likely to get the help you need.

You must, however, be sure to give the doctor the information he or she needs to understand your unique situation. There isn't another woman like you, so tell your own story, with all its details. Your daughters' too! Make sure your doctor knows your:

- Age

- Ethnicity

- Family history

- Medical history: PCOS, blood pressure (BP), blood glucose (BG), cholesterol (lipids)

- Lifestyle

- Physical activity level

- Pregnancy history

- Smoking habits

- Waist size

Resources

General Resources

May 12 has been named National Women's Check-Up Day. You can get free screenings for diabetes, breast cancer, heart disease, and other diseases. To find a center near you, go to: *www.4woman.gov/whw*

Associations

National Coalition of 100 Black Women
38 West 32nd Street
Suite 1610
New York, NY 10001
212-947-2196
www.ncbw.org/about/home.html

National Black Women's Health Project, Inc.
600 Pennsylvania Avenue, SE
Suite 310
Washington, D.C. 20003
202-543-4000
www.blackwomenshealth.org

Sisters Network, Inc.
8787 Woodway Drive
Suite 4207
Houston, TX 77063
866-781-1808
www.sistersnetworkinc.org

La Leche League International
PO Box 4079
Schaumburg, IL 60168-4079
847-519-7730
www.lalecheleague.org

Planned Parenthood Federation of America
810 7th Avenue
New York, NY 10019
800-230-7526
www.plannedparenthood.org

Pregnancy and Newborn Health Education Center
March of Dimes Birth Defects Foundation
1275 Mamaroneck Avenue
White Plains, NY 10605
888-MODIMES (888-663-4637)
www.marchofdimes.com

National Organization on Fetal Alcohol Syndrome (NOFAS)
216 G Street, NE
Washington, D.C. 20002
202-785-4585
www.nofas.org

National SAFE KIDS campaign
1301 Pennsylvania Avenue, NW, Suite 1000
Washington, D.C. 20004
202-662-0600
www.safekids.org

NIH Osteoporosis and Related Bone Diseases-National Resource Center
1232 22nd Street, NW
Washington, D.C. 20037-1292
800-624-2663
www.osteo.org

National Youth Violence Prevention Resource Center
8401 Colesville Road, Suite 200
Silver Spring, MD 20910
888-Safeyouth (888-723-3968)
www.SAFEYOUTH.org

Books and Magazines

Women's Bodies, Women's Wisdom: Creating Physical and Emotional Health and Healing, by Christiane Northrup, MD. Bantam Books, 1994.

Dr. Susan Love's Breast Book, by Susan Love, MD, with Karen Lindsey. Addison-Wesley Publishing Co., 1995.

The Osteoporosis Book: A Guide for Patients and Their Families, by Nancy E. Lane, MD. Oxford University Press, 1999.

101 Tips for a Healthy Pregnancy with Diabetes, by Patti B. Geil, MS, RD, CDE, and Laura B. Hieronymus, MSEd, APRN, CDE. American Diabetes Association, 2003.

The Nursing Mother's Companion, by Kathleen Huggins and Ruth A. Lawrence. National Book Network, 1999.

The Mother's Almanac, by Marguerite Kelly and Elia Parsons. Broadway Books, 1975, 1992.

The Mother's Almanac II, by Marguerite Kelly. Doubleday, 1989.

Different and Wonderful, by Dr. Darlene Powell Hopson and Dr. Derek S. Hopson. Prentice-Hall, 1990.

Six Weeks to Better Parenting, by Caryl W. Krueger. Pelican, 1981.

Teach Your Child to Behave, by Charles E. Shaefer, PhD, and Theresa Foy DiGeronimo. Plume, 1990.

Women & Diabetes, 2nd edition, by Laurinda M. Poirier, MPH, RN, CDE, and Katharine M. Coburn, MPH. American Diabetes Association, 2000.

SELF magazine. This magazine does an excellent job of providing variety and clear instruction in physical activity and good nutrition for women.

CHAPTER

12

MEN'S HEALTH

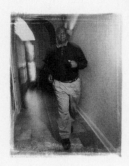

If you want to live a long, healthy life, develop a chronic disease and take good care of it.

—Mark Twain

I do hope that you are reading this chapter, even though it's usually the women in the family who buy the books. Men are more into action, I know. And that's good, because it is your actions that will make you a man to respect.

It is cool to lift weights and develop muscles in your arms and chest—to have a six-pack belly. It is cool to play basketball like Mike—or baseball or football like the athletes we all love to watch. Let me suggest that it's even cooler to find sports that follow you when you have to leave team sports behind. You may not realize it, but it is cool to eat well and wisely. Many of your favorite athletes are well aware of this fact. They also lift weights and some of them even take yoga classes for the flexibility it gives them.

It is not cool, however, to smoke and drink a lot of alcohol and to take recreational drugs. I don't think any of this comes as a surprise, but sometimes it helps to state the obvious. When kids copy this behavior because they see you do it, they are damaging their growing minds and bodies. Damage that we doctors may not be able to repair. The bottom line is that whatever you do shows up sooner or later in your face and your body. The sexiest man is the man who takes care of himself, so he looks good and feels good for 100 years. Isn't that a goal you could get behind?

Many teenage weight lifters, boxers, and athletes know what to do to be in top shape. If those years are behind you (or weren't ever there at all), you can adopt the healthy lifestyle suggested in this book right now. Let me put it this way, if you're at a point where sex is "not like it used to be," there is room for improvement. The choice is up to you.

In the Bedroom

Impotence or erectile dysfunction (ED) may be the health complication that you fear most and with good reason. High blood pressure and diabetes put you at higher risk for this complication. You can keep your blood vessels and nerves healthy with good nutrition, exercise, and using "healthy" ways to cope with stress. These are the tools you can use to prevent ED, if you want to. When you develop a health problem like high blood pressure or diabetes—and black men have the highest risks for these diseases—the blood vessels through which your blood circulates and the nerves that send traffic signals all over your body can be damaged—damaged enough to cause impotence.

If it happens, and if it happens more than once or twice, don't wait. Go to your doctor to try to find the cause. This is necessary. The earlier you take care of things the easier it is to fix. However, don't automatically assume that it's a physical problem. Often impotence is caused by emotional or psychological stress, which your doctor can help you with as well.

Your problems may be caused by a medication you are taking. High blood pressure medications, which you take to save yourself from a heart attack or stroke, have side effects that may affect your sex life. That's why it is important to try to control your blood pressure with exercise and good eating first. That way, even if you have to take medication, you can be taking the lowest dose possible.

A Wise Man Practices

Please practice safe sex for your own health and for the health of your partner—and any children of yours. If you think you have a sexually transmitted disease (STD), get treatment right away. Be responsible for what you do. The list of diseases that you and a sexual partner may be sharing, whether you know it or not, can be found on page 219.

Watch the Pressure

As a black man, you are more at risk of high blood pressure when you are under stress than anyone else. Research reported in the *American Journal of Hypertension* (June 1995) showed that the blood pressure of all the men and women in the study went up under stress. They had three stresses to deal with: making a public speech, adding numbers in their head, and having an ice pack held on their forehead. The men's blood vessels constricted more tightly than the women's, and the African American men had the most constriction of all. This may be why even our male children are more at risk of stroke than other children. The message is clear: You must find ways to deal with stress. You need to become aware of your tension, breathe deeply, and relax your muscles and your blood vessels. You may run a higher risk of hypertension and diabetes, but stopping to count to ten and breathing deeply may be more powerful for you than anyone else, too. Exercise, counseling, a change in attitude—all will help you relax yourself away from high blood pressure.

By the way, smoking is one of the worst things you can do for your sex life. It constricts your blood vessels, which is an action you don't need more of. Smoke has all sorts of toxic junk for your body, slipped in by way of your lungs that hand it over to your circulating blood. Quit smoking. If you're having trouble there are a variety of resources open to you—hypnosis, classes, the patch, gum, etc.

Exercise

Exercise lowers your blood pressure and your cholesterol, and reduces your body fat. It makes you feel good by easing stress, building muscles, and releasing endorphins—the feel-good hormones from the brain, some of which are more powerful than morphine. Exercise stimulates your nervous system and makes your heart stronger. It heightens your immune system. It's not the car you drive or the clothes you wear that make you a man. It's how much exercise you do every day. It's how well you take care of your body.

In this society, men are more likely than women to exercise. But depending on their age and outlook, a lot of men don't exercise the way they did when they were younger. That's too bad, because it seems like they wait until *after* they have a heart attack to start walking around and around the block. Why wait? Why not start walking today and pass up the experience of a heart attack?

The research is overwhelming on this point about men. If you walk 30 minutes a day, you cut your risk of type 2 diabetes by 30 to 40%. If you already have type 2 diabetes, you still get great benefits from walking. If you walk three to four hours a week—whether it's 30 minutes a day, or one-hour walks three days of the week—you cut your risk of dying of a heart attack almost in half. You don't have to go to the gym,

Walking Your Baby Back Home?
Researchers who studied thousands of men with type 2 diabetes found that men who walked the fastest were the least likely to die from any cause. The ones who walked briskly three to five hours a week reaped the greatest benefits for their hearts.

you don't have to wear lycra shorts, but you do have to get yourself out there every day—or most every day.

Just Get Going

Move fast enough to get your heart rate up, but not so fast you're too out of breath for a long conversation. Walk so you're doing something good for yourself and setting a good example for the folks around you—young and old. Be proud of yourself for this.

You can park at the far end of the parking lot and walk in. Besides, you're less likely to get the doors to your car dented way out there. Walking up the stairs instead of taking the elevator can help you lose three pounds a year. That doesn't sound like much, but it's sure better than putting on three pounds a year, which is what most people do!

I just can't stress the benefits of walking enough. And unlike pills, walking has no bad side effects. Walking is a good exercise for people with diabetes, with physical problems, and for the elderly. There are many research studies these days of the benefits of walking for the human body. And the results are overwhelmingly positive. Taking a walk can save your life and the lives of your family and friends. Walking helps lower body fat—especially in that middle section that we want to see go away—it raises your good cholesterol (HDL) levels, and makes your cells more sensitive to

My Role Model
On my drive home from work, I see an older gentleman walking. He is thin with iron gray hair, and from the extreme slant of his shoulders and body, you can see that he has had a stroke that affected his left side. He walks briskly, swinging the stiffened arm and leg. He walks in rain or sunshine, snow or wind—in all the weathers that the rest of us use as an excuse not to. Because I have passed him at various places along his route over the past three years, I know that he walks five miles every day. I know that he has not missed a day in three years. Perhaps the stroke gave him the reason to be so dedicated. Perhaps the long walk makes him calm, so he can sleep at night. Perhaps his wife is the kind of woman it is good to take a break from. Perhaps now she's gone, and he's walking off his grief. I don't know what motivates him, but he inspires me by his faithfulness and the results. Even after the stroke, he is one of the healthiest men I see.

insulin, which lowers your blood sugar levels. Walking helps lower your blood pressure without pills.

Know Your Syndrome X Risk

Are you at risk for Metabolic Syndrome, also called Syndrome X? The National Cholesterol Education Panel has condensed the risks to five easily checked factors:

1. Abdominal obesity (Is your waist bigger than 40 inches?)
2. High triglycerides (Found with a simple blood test)
3. Low HDL (good) cholesterol (blood test)
4. High fasting blood sugar (blood test)
5. High blood pressure

If you have three of the five risk factors, then you and your heart can benefit from some lifestyle changes right now. If you are a smoker, start there. The American Heart Association says that the research shows that people with heart disease who exercise have a lower death rate than those who don't.

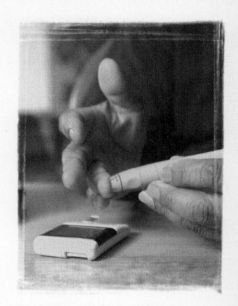

Stress Busters

You need to reduce your stress. Fortunately, there are several toolkits that you have available to you to relieve stress in your life. Exercise, losing weight, behavior change, sleep, hobbies, and getting organized are more powerful than you may know right now.

Exercise. The heart and blood vessels of active men respond less to stress. Working out puts stress on your body, so your heart and blood vessels are used to it and don't get excited. The feel-good brain chemicals released during exercise help handle stress, too. Exercises like tai chi, martial arts, and yoga all focus on stretching, strength, and breathing correctly. They can help you learn to slow down.

Lose weight. A combination of losing some weight and exercising regularly helps make your heart and blood vessels calmer under stress.

Counseling. See a counselor who does cognitive or behavioral therapy. This short-term therapy focuses on problem ideas and behaviors and helps you change your responses to those stress triggers.

Sleep. Get at least 8 hours of sleep a night. If you snore and wake up feeling groggy and tired, you may have sleep apnea. See a doctor for help getting the rest you need.

Hobbies and activities you enjoy. Make time for yourself to be quiet and creative. Find things you like to do.

Organization. Slow down. Bring some energy back home and get yourself organized to meet the day. Cleaning up the clutter in your closet and in your daily life will relieve some of the stress on you.

Make the Most of It

Do Something Creative

Doing something creative—being a maker, not a breaker—is another key to good health. There is plenty to do, including helping the children learn, cleaning up the community, building playgrounds, and starting a community garden. There are opportunities for growth and generosity in every community. Look around yours and start giving of yourself. Few things do more for your health—emotional, spiritual, and physical—than being creative and helping others.

Read More

You need to be literate. Read books. Help others learn to read, too. In this world, you can be healthier if you can read. You need to be able to read books, magazines, newspapers, and health information on the Internet.

Take Responsibility for Yourself

If you are a father, be a responsible man they can look up to. Do what you can to avoid having children until you are ready and able to care for them. Find out what the legal, financial, and emotional responsibilities of a father are. Find a role model. If you do have children, get connected with them. Read to them. If you don't have any children, you can volunteer to read to kids at a local shelter or in a Head Start class. Get involved in the lives of the children around you, and you will be a rich man.

Franklyn M. Malone, founder of the Alexandria Family Learning Resource Center in northern Virginia, noted, "One of the most important aspects of a child's life is a positive interaction with a father figure. Dads often hold the key to their children's success. We have to put dads back where they belong as being responsible for their children."

Whether or not you are a dad, you can make a difference in the lives of all the children in your neighborhood. Step up to the plate and hit some home runs in this ballpark, if you will.

Resources

Online

The nonprofit Men's Health Network offers free or discounted screenings for diabetes, prostate cancer, and high blood pressure. Check for sites near you at:
www.menshealth.org

100 Black Men is an organization of African American men dedicated to improving their communities by focusing on business opportunities and education for the children and anyone else who wants it. Check out their website:
www.100blackmen.com

The pro basketball player Bill Russell works with a program of men sharing what they know with children and teens. Find out more at:
www.mentoring.org

and
www.helpyourcommunity.org

Tomorrows Black Men is a nonprofit organization that works with at-risk young black males to raise their standard of living and improve the quality of life for their families and communities. Visit their website at:
www.tomorrowsblackmen.org

Associations

CDC National Prevention Information Network (HIV/AIDS, STDs, TB)
P.O. Box 6003
Rockville, MD 20849-6003
800-458-5231
www.cdcnpin.org

HIV/AIDS Treatment Information Center
P.O. Box 6303
Rockville, MD 20849-6303
800-448-0440
www.hivatis.org

**National Clearinghouse for Alcohol
and Drug Information**
P.O. Box 2345
Rockville, MD 20847-2345
800-729-6686
www.health.org

Center for Minority Veterans
810 Vermont Avenue, NW
Washington, D.C. 20420
800-827-1000
www.va.gov

Magazines

Men's Health magazine is on newsstands and online at:
www.menshealth.com

CHAPTER

13

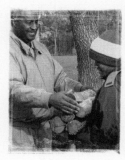

BECOMING
AN ELDER

When you think about it, growing older is actually something everyone wants to do—isn't it? Why else is good health so important? Still, you don't really want to be thought of as old, do you? There seems to be a line into old age that no one in America wants to cross. That may be because of an unfortunate image of old age as a time of frailty and weakness. What is that old saying? The one about the wisdom and cunning of old age overcoming the strength and advantages of youth?

I am sure you can remember family members and friends who were hale and hearty right into their 90s. Folks who were quick, intelligent, loving, and funny. Folks who were pretty healthy, too. Because of their long lives and experiences, you could take a problem to them and get a new perspective on what to do. These elders were able to take trips with the family, whether to the local museum or on an airplane far away. Able to cook dinner every night (and better than anyone else in the family). I am sure that every one of us wants to be that sort of an elder—loved, valued, included, and most important, contributing to the family and the community right up to the transition to another world. How are you doing so far?

There are, once again, things that you can do to achieve the goal of wise, hearty old age. You can do things for the physical part of you and things for the spiritual, emotional, and mental parts of you. They're all connected, so helping one area helps all areas of your life. If you start eating well and exercising daily—including stretching and lifting those two-pound bags of rice twice a week—you are paying into the only real insurance there is for healthy old age. Exercise makes your body stronger, more flexible, energized, and relaxed. It is the only known intervention that can slow your physiological aging process. A sedentary lifestyle, on the other hand, ages you more quickly.

Ignore the 30-somethings who say humans lose strength and physical ability with every passing decade. Research at Tufts University conducted by Dr. William Evans showed that 80-somethings and 90-somethings, even those in nursing homes, can start weight exercises and triple their muscle strength and add new muscle mass in two months time. Exercise is good for you every day of your life. Don't ever stop.

To keep the spirit, emotion, and mind parts of you healthy, exercising actually helps—and requires—a mental and spiritual dedication to your goals. If you respect your body and feel grateful for the miraculous things it can do, you are much more likely to be physically active and well. As a guideline for the spiritual, mental, emotional part of you, try to be a "maker" not a "breaker." There are activities you can start now:

- Love the folks around you

- Share in a spirit-based community like your local church

- Find ways that you can make your community a better place to grow up

The point is you are never too old to do meaningful work, to do good deeds, or to lend a helping hand.

Multiple Medications

The fact is that diseases and chronic conditions will progress despite following the best exercise and meal plans. If this should happen to you, please comfort yourself with knowing that you have needed less medication all these years because of your efforts. If you are now taking medications, talk with your doctor about them at every visit, especially if you see several different doctors. An emergency room visit could get you on a drug that your regular doctor does not know about. Take all your medications with you to each appointment in a bag. See if you still need them all. See if you could take a lower dose of any of them. As people age, they tend to need smaller doses of their medications.

Often doctors require the most complicated drug schedule of the group least likely to be able to follow it—either because of mental confusion or poverty. Both of which, ironically, can actually be caused by the interaction of too many prescription drugs. Many people in this category are elderly. Before you get there, do all you can to stay healthy so you don't need to take many different drugs. To keep from getting confused or overwhelmed, ask your doctor for a simple drug schedule that will work for you. Get yourself one of those plastic pill organizers. It really helps you remember whether you took your pill or not. If you have recently had a serious illness and are taking several new drugs for awhile, ask the doctor or nurse to draw you a chart so you can see how many medications you are taking each day, when you take them, and why you take them. If the pill bottles all look alike—and even if they don't—it might be wise to mark each one with a bright color, so you know which one you're picking up. Accidentally taking a medication three times a day instead of once a day can get you a quick trip to the hospital. Don't be afraid to ask a trusted friend or nurse to put your medications in a weekly pill box for you.

One sure way to stay healthier while you are taking medication is to drink enough water every day. Ask your doctor how much water you should be drinking. Some conditions, such as kidney disease and high blood pressure, may require that you drink only certain amounts of water.

Help with the Cost of Your Prescriptions

If you are on Medicare* and don't have insurance for drugs, and your income is under $28,000 a year ($38,000 as a couple), there is a program to help pay for your prescriptions. Actually, there are about 240 programs to help people of all ages with the cost of their prescription drugs, but where do you and the 10 million other folks who need them find out more? The National Council on the Aging has a web site, *www.benefitscheckuprx.org*, listing all the programs, including 30 state-funded pharmacy programs. Drug companies also have assistance programs (about 120 right now) and for many of these programs there are no age or income requirements. It never hurts to ask. On the site are also drug-discount cards, which are free to consumers and must provide at least a 20% discount.

Before you log onto BenefitsCheckUpRx, gather the pill bottles, or those of the relative or friend you are helping, and make a list of all the drugs you need. Also find bank statements to establish your monthly and yearly income. Then you

---

* All claims about Medicare are based upon information available at the time of this printing. Medicare legislation is constantly changing. To get current information on Medicare benefits and programs visit *www.medicare.gov* or call 1-800-MEDICARE (1-800-633-4227).

are ready to answer any questions. There is a pull-down list of drug names, but you want to be sure you're getting the right ones, so double-check your spelling. Some drugs have similar names but do very different things to your body. You don't have to know the name of the drug manufacturer, the website does that for you. You will receive a report of the programs for which you qualify and information for how to apply.

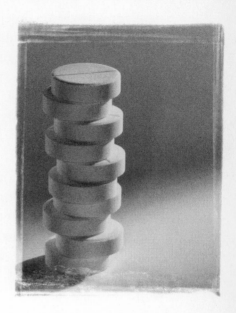

Other Cost Saving Methods for Prescription Drugs

- Consider a mail-order or online pharmacy. If you do decide to buy from an Internet pharmacy, please read the guidelines for doing so safely on page 30. If you have a prescription like insulin that needs to be refrigerated or protected from extremes of temperature, ask what the company does to protect the shipment to you.

- Ask your doctor if you could have a generic drug instead of a brand name, because they are just as safe and effective, but less expensive.

- Ask if you could have a larger number of pills if buying in quantity is less expensive.

- Ask your doctor if your medication could be split in two. Some drugs can be split, some cannot. Generally, pills with a line scored in the top can be split; capsules cannot. If your pills can be split, you could get a prescription for a higher dose and then cut the pills in two to get your dose. You get two pills for the price of one. Take care to get even halves. You can buy an inexpensive pill cutter at the drug store to help you.

● Check around to see if there is a Medicare HMO in your area. You usually pay only a small co-payment for your prescriptions.

● If you are a member of an organization such as AARP (American Association of Retired People), check to see if they offer a discount prescription drug program. AARP does; it's called MemberRx Choice (go to *www.aarppharmacy.com* or call 1-800-439-4457).

● If you are a military veteran and you get health care at a local Veterans or military hospital, you know that your drugs are covered. There is sometimes a small co-payment. Veterans of WWII and Korea are eligible for a program called TriCare for Life, which covers all drug costs. Younger veterans can get prescription drugs by mail order for $9 a prescription.

● You can also skip the Internet and call your local area agency on aging. To find that number call the Eldercare Locator at 1-800-677-1116. They can match your age and financial information with programs that can assist you. They can even check BenefitsCheckUpRx for you!

● Whatever route you choose, be an informed buyer. Compare prices at your corner drug store, a big chain drugstore, mail-order drug stores, and Internet drug stores. Many pharmacies already have senior discounts or frequent shopper discounts that you probably qualify for.

Things to Check in Your Insurance Coverage
• Deductible (how much you pay before insurance starts) • Co-payment (what part of the bills you must pay) • Preexisting Condition (how long you must wait before insurance covers you for diabetes or any disease that you already have) • Limit to what you must pay each year • Limit to what the insurance company will pay in a lifetime • Coverage for diabetes care and supplies or other care you need • Whether you choose your own doctor or use those in the system Adapted from *Right from the Start*, American Diabetes Association, 2003.

Insurance Questions

If you need help getting insurance or finding out what is available to you, you can call your State Insurance Commissioner's office. Look under State Government in the blue pages of the phone book. If you have problems with insurance, call the National Insurance Consumer Hotline at 1-800-942-4242.

Acting on Behalf of Another Person

If you are taking care of someone, help both the patient and the doctor cover all the areas that may affect his or her health. The doctor needs to know:

- Who does the shopping for the elder person?
- Who cooks?

- Can he swallow pills?

- Can she afford her medications?

- Can he see?

- Can she understand the label?

- Which other drugs does he take that might interact with each other and cause problems?

If the patient is to take drugs to lower blood pressure, be sure the dose is small enough that it is lowered gradually, so she doesn't fall.

Remember that it is easier for elderly people to get dehydrated. They generally don't feel thirsty, even as they are getting dehydrated. Ask the doctor if it's okay to get a pitcher, fill it each morning, and get a good number of daily glasses of water. Dehydration should be taken very seriously; it not only increases the effect of their medications, it can even be deadly. Dehydration and high blood sugar is a dangerous combination that can lead to coma and possibly death. This condition, called hyperosmolar hyperglycemic state (HHS), occurs most often in elderly people in nursing homes who have diabetes. Ask the nursing home staff to be sure that the patient drinks enough water every day and to check her blood sugar at least once a day. People aged 80 or older should not take metformin for diabetes, and long acting sulfonylureas (chlorpropramide) can be dangerous for them, too.

Living Wills and the Like

The doctor should bring up the topic of living wills and caretaker issues, ideally while the person in question is able to make these decisions for himself. These discussions may take weeks or months. Ask the doctor to explain what a do not resuscitate (DNR) order means, especially if a terminal illness is involved. Write down the patient's wishes and what level of care is wanted.

Look at What Is Happening

The caregiver and doctor need to look at the patient's situation closely. Can she afford treatment? Why is he making this decision? Can she exercise? Does he know what healthy food choices are?

Hospitals and nursing homes do not necessarily provide healthy meals. You may need to get involved here, just like you've gotten involved in the school lunch programs at school. Wouldn't it be wonderful if the local nursing home residents grew their own garden and helped prepare their meals, too? Many of them have the skills that would make both programs flourish—and would keep them healthier and happier, too.

How tight should her blood glucose control be? What are his other health problems? Elderly folks are more likely to have several problems. For example, a visit to the ophthalmologist may turn up glaucoma, cataract, and macular degeneration in the same patient.

Is she still mentally able to manage her medications and self-care? As caregiver you need to double-check what the patient is telling the doctor. And what the doctor tells the patient. Having another set of ears and eyes is valuable in these exchanges.

The elderly are at increased risk for depression. Especially if all they have to do is watch TV. Watch for these symptoms:

- Difficulty sleeping

- Not eating

- Not doing activities that they used to enjoy

- Refusing to see friends or to go out

- Feeling sad and blue

- Thinking of suicide

See a doctor for evaluation and, perhaps, a prescription. Be sure that they are drinking enough water every day. Good nutrition—those fruits, vegetables, and whole grains again—and being active every day, especially outside in fresh air, makes a world of difference in a person's mental state. Also, depression could be a side effect of the mix of medications that they are already taking. Ask the doctor about that possibility, too.

There are several gentle body therapies that help folks of all ages, but may be especially comforting to an elder. Massage heals by restoring circulation and easing muscle tension and pain, but it also provides the touching that we all need in order to be healthy.

Acupuncture is an ancient (more than 3,000 years old) treatment for pain and other chronic symptoms. While there are still ongoing studies as to the effectiveness of acupuncture, there have been some promising results in terms of pain treatment. Once again, it never hurts to try and you have only benefits to gain.

To Age Wisely

To keep your mind as active as your body, you may want to go to school. My 83-year-old aunt was not home when I called to wish her a happy birthday. She was at an aerobics class at the local community college. She had taken courses in history there the year before. She has had a long, not particularly easy life. She was a flapper in the 20s, lived through the depression, had two children, a difficult husband, and never much money. But she has always been delighted to see us and ready to sing and laugh. She has an interest in the world around her that is undiminished by time, and her experiences have gifted her with the ability to make wise observations. If you don't have any examples of wise elders in your life, why not become one? Live every day. Use what you have learned from the past to make your own life happier and healthier, and to improve the lives of those around you.

Learn to read or wake up your reading skills. Reading to your own kids or grandkids or to the kids at a local shelter is a gift for you all. You might ask at the library about free classes in reading. Or ask if they have videos on reading. Your local library or adult learning center (often in the high school) may have videos for you to check out for free.

You might take up bridge or chess, games that are known to sharpen your mind. You might join a book club and enter into discussions of the book and the wider world. You might start an elder club to discuss neighborhood and community issues, and see where you might help. You might all write your elected representatives to tell them what your community needs. You can volunteer your help at schools, at hospitals, at community centers. Your example teaches others how to be in this world. Your voice counts. Please use it for the highest good of all concerned. This is why we need our elders.

Resources

Online

Go to the National Council on the Aging website at:
www.ncoa.org

To check on all the available drug assistance programs look at BenefitsCheckUpRx:
www.benefitscheckup.org

Look into free and low-cost prescription drugs and apply for a free discount card to save up to 25% on drugs at:
www.institute-dc.org

To contact your local representatives in Congress go to:
www.congress.org

Associations

American Association of Retired People (AARP)
Inexpensive AARP membership provides discounts, services, and savings, a bi-monthly magazine, and bulletin. A discount prescription program called MemberRx Choice, which is accepted at many pharmacies, costs $19.95 a year.
800-424-3410
TTY 877-434-7598
www.aarp.org

BAM! Body and Mind
Centers for Disease Control and Prevention
1600 Clifton Road, NE
MSC-04
Atlanta, GA 30333
800-311-3435
www.bam.gov

The Congress of National Black Churches
2000 L Street, NW
Suite 225
Washington, D.C. 20036
202-296-5657
www.cnbc.org

National Caucus and Center on Black Aged, Inc.
1220 L Street, NW
Suite 800
Washington, D.C. 20005
202-637-8400
www.ncba-aged.org

Books

From Age-ing to Sage-ing, by Rabbi Zalman Schachter-Shalomi and Ronald S. Miller. Warner Books, 1995.

How to Save Up to $3,000 on Your Diabetes Expenses, by Leslie Dawson. American Diabetes Association, 2004.

14

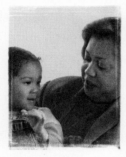

> *There are those who make things happen. There are those who watch things happen. And there are those who sit around and wonder what the hell happened.*
>
> **—Woody Allen**

HOPE FOR THE FUTURE

Yours, Mine, and the Children's

Sometimes it feels like a lot of us have resigned ourselves to doom. We look at our parents and our grandparents and say, "Why bother? I'm just going to end up the same way." We tell ourselves that taking care of a chronic condition like diabetes or heart disease isn't worth the effort. We resign ourselves to mediocre health. We tell ourselves there's no hope.

Well, I'm going to tell you something: There is hope. There is much that you can do. There is much that your health "consultants" can do. Small acts from each of us every day translate to hope and miraculous outcomes. We can extend our lives and our quality of life more than ever before. We can spend more time on this earth with the people we love.

So ask yourself: What are your goals? Do you know what you need to do to get there?

Health Insurance? Insure with Wellness

You may lament that your health insurance doesn't cover all the care that you need. You may lament that you don't have health insurance. You surely lament how long it takes to fill out the paperwork for insurance coverage. These are serious problems, but please think about what I am saying before you despair. You can change your own health for the better, and you can do it with the choices that you make everyday about what to eat and how active you are. These choices are free, and they are also priceless in their importance in your life and the lives of your children.

Being well saves you money. Saves your life. Having a lot of people be well saves the healthcare system from crashing down around us. We want it to be there when we need it. Let us all have a "health and wellness" agenda as the number one priority in our lives. Remember the old saying: If you don't have your health, you don't have anything?

In many ways we are challenged to flip our health care system right-side up. Currently we are spending an awful lot of money on highly specialized care, on advanced-stage diseases, or on end-of-life care. Conversely, we spend very little on prevention, early detection, or robust health and wellness agendas. The current system of health care is literally upside down!

Insure your health by doing the things that you know will help, like eating good food and exercising every day. Smile. Learn how to let stress roll off your back. Stop smoking. Learn how to build something or paint something or cook something or grow something in a garden. Do creative acts every day.

Turn off the television set. Go make a reality show of your own. Even if you're the only one watching, you're the most important viewer.

You Need to Read

There are some wonderful toolkits for us out there. I want you, your parents, and your children to be able to find them and to use them, so we need to read. In this world, we all need to be able to read and to understand what we read. Literacy is the key to good health—regular literacy, health and medical literacy, and computer literacy. Be an information seeker.

Now there are some folks who haven't yet learned to read, but they keep themselves from doing it because they feel embarrassed. They need to feel a passion for reading. There is real power in being able to read. I want everyone to be able to read everything from food labels on cereal boxes to the Declaration of Independence.

It might help if we do away with some myths about poor readers. Poor readers are not stupid, they just haven't learned to read—yet. Or they're no longer able to see well or perhaps think clearly. Poor readers can be found at every economic level. You can have a job and not be able to read. Poor readers are not necessarily poor. You see? The only bad thing about poor reading is that it keeps you from getting where you want to go.

There are some excellent videos and audiotapes that can help people on a quest to become literate. If you know someone who cannot read or your children cannot read well, tell them about those tapes. People who listen to a book on tape and follow along in their own book can improve their reading exponentially. Get creative, because reading is fun.

Gardens and the Community

Children eat what they are served. Wouldn't it be wonderful to serve them food fresh from the garden? Many of us live in urban areas, and our children grow up without seeing or par-

Where and What We Need to Change

Again, let me encourage you to lift your voice and use your energy to get involved in turning back the unhealthy tide in this country. Start with your own family and we'll all help each other succeed.

Where	Change
School	Return to good nutrition and PE.
Workplace	Ask for better food choices and exercise opportunities.
Community	Create safe parks, playgrounds, bike paths, and programs for everyone.
Health care	Make sure insurance covers education and regular check-ups, things that keep us well.
Government	Regulate the food industry and don't target the children.
Home	Make healthy behavior changes.
Nursery	Start breastfeeding to prevent type 1 and type 2 diabetes.

ticipating in the cycles of life. It means much more to watch corn ripen and get to eat it fresh from the stalk than to buy it at the grocery store. Gardens can brighten empty lots and fire escapes and rooftops on every block in every city. Following are some examples of successful gardening projects that were gathered by Laurel Kallenbach for the March/April 2003 edition of *Yoga Journal*.

A group that encourages new gardens and saves established ones in New York City is called the Green Guerillas. They work to preserve garden spaces where all members of the community can come together—a safe place for kids and elders. You can learn more about them at *www.greengueril-las.org*. In the past 20 years, flower, herb, and vegetable gardens have popped up in cities all around the country. They provide healthy produce for families and for enterprising teens to sell to local restaurants. Gardens can thrive in inner cities and help the residents thrive, too.

It doesn't take much imagination to see that the most successful food programs would be in schools that have their own gardens. Kids learn many lessons in the garden and from growing the food that they also prepare in the school kitchen. Students at Martin Luther King Jr. School in Berkeley, California, for example, show the rest of us just how successful this type of project can be. The Edible Schoolyard was started by a famous chef named Alice Waters. Learn more about it at *www.edibleschoolyard.org*.

Another successful story of kids in the garden was described in *Newsweek* magazine (see below) about the Ecology-Technology Academy in inner city Philadelphia, where every kid qualifies for the Free Lunch Program. Marvin Galvin, founder of the garden program, decided the school should cultivate a taste for healthy foods in every school. All subjects in the school curriculum center on the one-acre garden, which even has fruit trees. During the summer, the kids invite parents in to eat the healthy meals they have learned to cook. Students also get to sell excess produce at a local farm stand. This is a long way from eating fast food three or four nights a week.

In other schools, local chefs come in to the school to show both the lunchroom cooks and the kids better food choices and preparation techniques. The chefs show up at math class and talk about measuring ingredients. They go to the science classes and show how baking a cake can turn into a chemistry experiment.

Colorado State University's (CSU) food science and human nutrition department has developed a powerful new elementary school program aimed at second-graders called Program ENERGY. The goal is to get kids to change their behaviors to reach healthy weights and avoid type 2 diabetes. The students go home and involve their parents in new lifestyle choices, too. Program ENERGY uses science and math to teach kids how exercise and good nutrition make their bodies healthier. Classroom visits from a chef, a nurse, and a cultural anthropologist fueled interest in science games, growing plants, sugar investigation, energy balance, and healthy snacks. Exercise was measured by steps on pedometers and by logging miles, the final walking goal being the distance from CSU to Disney World in Florida.

Program ENERGY is funded by the National Center for Research Resources at the National Institutes of Health (NIH), and is a partnership of community and university that includes scientists, teachers, health care professionals, farmers, and chefs. At the beginning and end of the program, the following areas were measured:

- Weight

- Waist

- Circumference

- Health and science knowledge

- Attitudes

- Behavior (using the pedometers)

It was clear that the children learned new behaviors and put them into practice. Most of them enjoyed doing so. The kids took home colorful one-page handouts to their parents every week to tell them about diabetes and how to prevent it. Students also took home a weekly family challenge to increase activity and diabetes knowledge. Students earned points when their families completed the challenges. Reports from the parents showed their better understanding of diabetes and that their time spent walking was twice as long as before. Your community may want to try this program, too.

Bloom Where You're Planted

If a garden can enrich and engage the youngsters in our communities, think what it could do for the elderly residents of nursing homes. If they could grow their own flower and vegetable gardens and help prepare the food, they would feel more involved and more independent. Their skills in gardening could also be passed on to local youngsters who need to learn them.

Gardeners of all ages might want to follow the example set by the Garden Writers of America. They started a project called Plant a Row for the Hungry (PAR) to encourage gardeners to share a portion of their produce with local soup kitchens and food banks. More than a million pounds of produce are donated every year. To learn more about PAR, contact *www.gwaa.org*.

Community Efforts at Exercise

You begin to see that if a community works together on a challenge, everyone gets to benefit from the work they do. Look at these examples of community-led health programs and follow their lead to make your community a healthier one.

In the Daycare

A health promotion in Regina, Canada, focused on getting the community involved in better nutrition and exercise. In a three-year project, a daycare center operated a community kitchen for parents to come and learn how to cook healthier meals. Volunteers also taught parents how to use the exercise equipment at the local recreation center. Community support helped the project succeed, said Jan Ayer, health-promotions manager there. People were more willing to workout with a buddy, and more salads are showing up at local feasts instead of a table full of desserts.

Yoga in the Classroom?

In San Francisco inner-city schools, a dedicated yoga teacher, Tony Sanchez, and his wife, Sandy Wong-Sanchez, are teaching elementary and middle-school teachers to use yoga stretches in the classroom. They don't wait until P.E. time either. Stretching happens whenever students are restless or unable to focus.

After working with teachers and students to see how yoga could help in the classroom, Tony developed the ABC Yoga Series, three 10-minute sets of stretches that improve balance, strength, flexibility, and concentration, and relieve stress. The teachers say it works. Before tests and whenever the students are nervous or fidgety, the teachers find that 5 or 10 minutes of yoga works wonders to calm and focus the students on learning.

Sandy went on to develop the Yoga Science Box, which contains 40 lesson plans for teachers to link yoga to subjects such as geometry, anatomy, physics, and health. Weaving all of these subjects into something that helps kids stay physically fit is an effort that is good for body and mind. Kids gain a whole new appreciation for their own bodies and how to make them work correctly.

One supporter of yoga in the schools is Gloria Siech, a content specialist in K-12 physical education in San Francisco. In an article in *Yoga Journal,* December 2002, she is quoted by Michael Castleman as saying, "Yoga is invaluable in the schools. It provides a good workout that develops flexibility, strength, and stamina. And it helps kids relax, settle down, and concentrate on academics—especially kids who are stressed because they're poor, don't speak good English, or have other serious challenges in their lives." Being creative and resourceful is the way to take control of your life, young and old.

For more information about the ABC Yoga Series visit *www.usyoga.org.* There you can also learn about the Yogasthma program, a seven-step program using yoga and breathing techniques to help kids control their asthma.

An article called "Helping Kids Get Fit" by Peg Tyre and others in the September 22, 2003, issue of *Newsweek* magazine listed some community efforts that were succeeding. You might go to a library, find this issue, and take inspiration from one of these school or church groups to make some healthy change in your own community.

After-School Activities

In Santa Ana, California, at Roosevelt Elementary School, a community group called Latino Health Access started a new kind of after-school program. Every day kids do exercises like sit-ups and jumping jacks, play sports, run an obstacle course, and learn better food choices with 5-a-Day (you guessed it, vegetables) Bingo. The LHA teaches educators activities for their students to engage in during recess so the kids come in refreshed and ready to study. They also started an exercise program for moms in the cafeteria in the morning.

Divine Meal Plans

It's not just schools taking up the fight against poor health and obesity. Pastor Donald Anthony grew concerned when he saw that his flock was being hit hard by heart disease, stroke, and diabetes at the same time that their waistlines were growing. He realized that these diseases could be controlled with diet and exercise, and he wanted to get started before the children began to suffer, too. The church ladies wrote and published a low-fat, low-salt cookbook, and put the new recipes in use after church and choir practice. Healthy snacks like veggies and dip replaced cookies and barbecued ribs. The congregation has come together to celebrate the gift of having a human body and to accept the responsibility to take better care of this gift.

Spread the Word

Take inspiration from these programs and make one to fit your community and the needs of the people in it. It is the only way we can take back our children's health. And along the way, restore our own. We need to develop strategies to prevent obesity and diabetes. Let's call it Prevent Dia-besity

We need to educate people about better health and how to get there. We need to help people change their behavior, whether it's finding something healthier to eat instead of fast food every day or finding a place to take a walk.

We are going to have to change the environment. We need to improve the school and the home environment, and the neighborhood, too! Don't be afraid to come up with ideas for ways to make healthy changes and to ask for them. Communities can get more use out of schools, parks, libraries, and organizations if they are used to educate both children and adults and to provide them safe places to learn and exercise.

You may not realize it but the vending machines at work are just as bad for you as they are for your kids at school. You want healthy choices in the machines, so when you forgot your lunch, you can choose fresh fruit and yogurt instead of a cola and candy bar.

It would be great if every business could offer a wellness program, but smaller companies may need you to come up with the idea for a walking club at lunch. You could invite

Weight Watchers to start a program onsite if no one can come and teach you about healthy meal planning. You might ask your human resources department if your health insurance coverage would support wellness programs or reimburse nutrition education for people with diabetes or heart disease. Show that you are concerned and involved. Ask for help to stay well. Ask for five-minute breaks each hour to stand up and stretch or to take a trip up and down the stairs. A short walk or some stretching helps you focus just as well as it does for the kids.

As Fran Kaufman, MD, past president of the American Diabetes Association and a pediatric endocrinologist in Los Angeles, would tell you, "If you want the vending machines out of the schools, you're going to have to go talk to the state legislators." She did. It took three years of visiting the state legislature in Sacramento, but the vending machines are going. The policies and funding of government agencies, whether they are local, state, or federal will have an effect on how healthy our communities are. And your dedication to getting your elected representatives to focus on issues that are important to you and your children will pay off. It helps if the whole community is writing letters, too.

We even need to start making our buildings healthier, too. The new Center for Disease Control (CDC) building going up in Atlanta has wide stairs front and center, and the elevators are hidden in the back. This invites people to walk and climb instead of stand and push buttons. Simple things like this can make a big difference. Let us think about how healthy communities look and then go create one.

The Beginning or the End?

The World Health Organization (WHO) announced in March 2003 that poor diet and no exercise has led to the epidemic in

heart disease, diabetes, osteoporosis, and cancer around the
world. By the year 2020, these chronic diseases will contribute to 75% of deaths worldwide.

Wouldn't you like to be part of the solution to this worldwide problem? Right now you have a golden opportunity to
do your best for yourself, your family, your friends, and your
local schools. This would lead directly to improvements in
your city, your country, and the whole wide world. I think
you may never find a job to do that is better than that.

INDEX